Tiny
Tastebuds

NATALIE PEALL

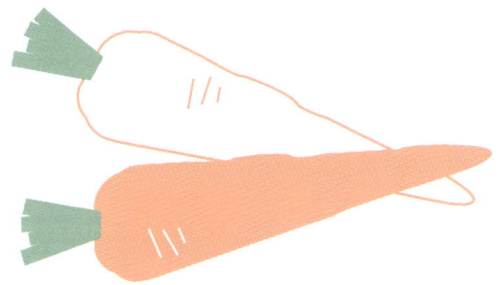

Tiny
Tastebuds

NATALIE PEALL

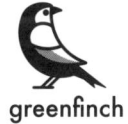

greenfinch

CONTENTS

RECIPE KNOW-HOW 83

RISE & SHINE 97

YUMMY LUNCHES 121

NO-FUSS DINNERS 143

TINY BITES & TREATS 164

FREEZER STASH 187

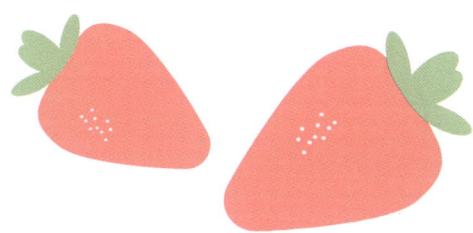

FOREWORD

When you become a parent, you're thrown into a whole new world of 'news'. While eating is something inherently familiar to us as adults, when it comes to feeding children, parents feel huge pressure to 'get it right'. With the rise of social media, forums, experts and resources, there has probably never been a time of more nutrition noise for parents to wade through when it comes to feeding their children.

Having worked with parents for over 14 years, and guided all ranges of feeding journeys, I know that parents universally recognize that starting solids is a time to establish healthy feeding foundations, paving the way to a long-term good relationship with food. But with this recognition of importance often comes trepidation, excitement, nervousness, desire for information and the inevitable late-night googling.

The desire to get a child's journey into food off to a flying start is backed by science. It is widely recognized that the first 1,000 days of a child's life (from conception to their second birthday) is a key window of opportunity to establish lifelong healthy eating habits. During this critical period, infants' taste preferences, eating patterns and even later health outcomes can be influenced by the foods they are introduced to.

More than ever, I believe parents want to make informed choices that feel aligned to their parenting style and are backed by science and a dose of real-life experience. This is where *Tiny Tastebuds* comes in, with plenty of information about baby-led weaning (BLW) but also (and arguably most importantly), the recipes, ideas and moral support to help you with the implementation! This book is the village every parent needs to support the start and onward journey of their child's love of food.

Tiny Tastebuds embraces the principles of baby-led weaning, empowering parents and caregivers to nurture their child's natural curiosity and autonomy when it comes to food. The book is a celebration of this approach, offering delicious and nutritious recipes tailored to support your little one's tiny tastebuds when exploring flavours and textures, while also making mealtimes an enjoyable experience for the whole family. Natalie weaves together science and information with relatable real-life experience – a combination that will help set you and your baby up for every success in your journey.

Natalie's recipes are not only vibrant and delicious, but accessible and practical – a factor that I appreciate more than ever since becoming a mum myself. As a huge advocate of eating with your family, this book also ensures that family-style eating and cooking one meal (not four) is at the heart of creating memorable moments around the table. Natalie's approach encourages inclusivity and togetherness (with factors like food allergies also taken into account), fostering a positive relationship with food for both parents and children alike. With her guidance, you'll discover the joy of cooking meals for your family and the satisfaction of nourishing your children with her wholesome, homemade dishes.

From one mum to another, I trust that you'll find as much delight in reading, digesting and savouring this book as I have.

Lucy Upton
The Children's Dietitian
Specialist Paediatric Dietitian and
Feeding Therapist

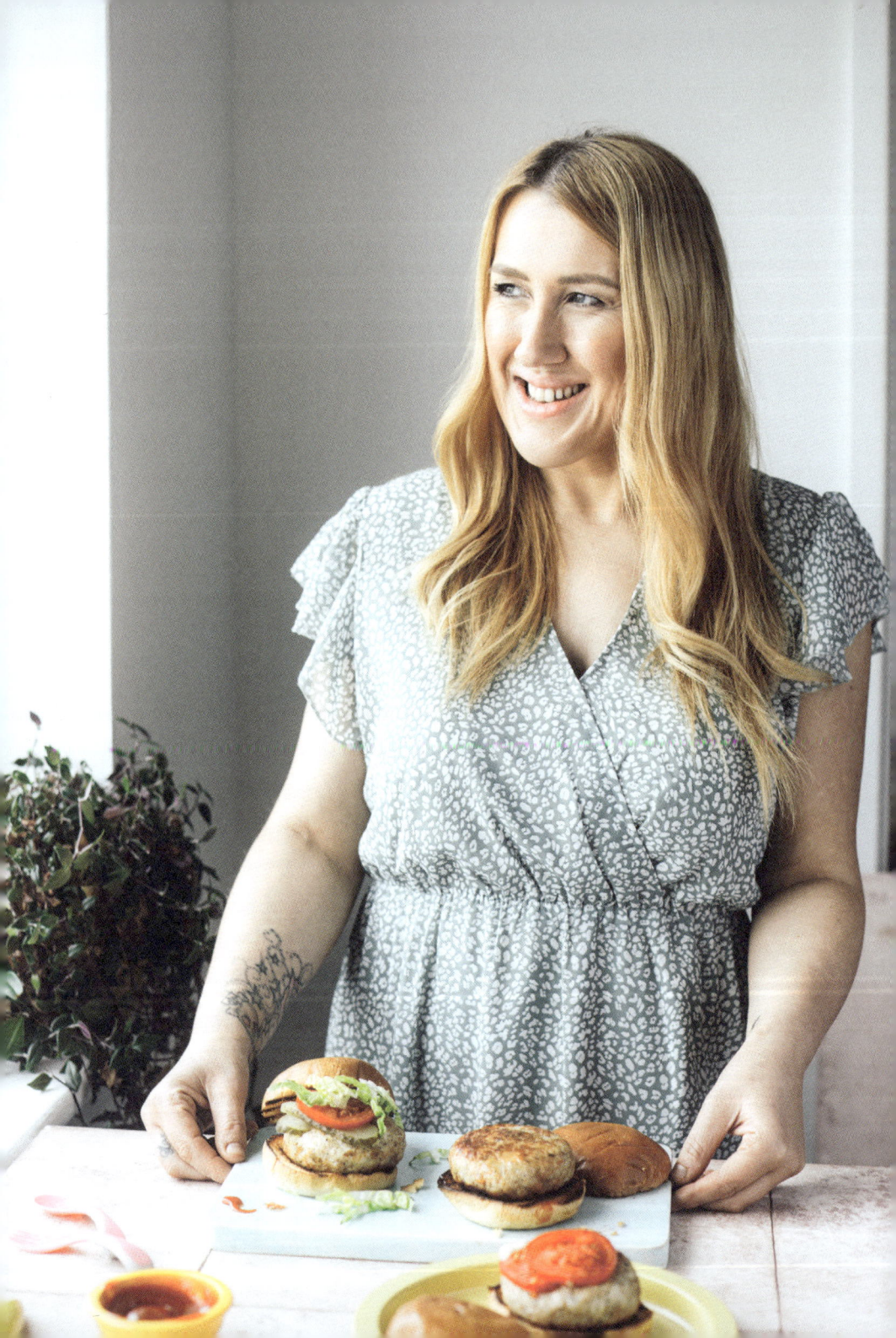

Hi, I'm Natalie.

I'm a mother of three, home cook and baby-led weaning (BLW) expert. I live in the Kent countryside in England with my ever-supportive husband, Steve, our wonderfully creative daughter, Annabelle, cheeky twin boys, Alex and Oliver, and two fluffy Persian cats. Family life is a whirlwind, constantly brimming with excitement and a bucket load of juggling!

The journey to this book began following Annabelle's birth. As she was coming up to six months old, I couldn't help but notice the glaring absence of weaning support. I was handed a leaflet and expected to know what I was doing. It's interesting that when you become a parent, you are often expected to know what to do, even though there is no school or university to equip you with the skills.

This grave lack of weaning support concerned me, given that this phase plays a pivotal role in a baby's development, and in establishing a healthy relationship with food. To add to the challenge, Annabelle grappled with a cow's milk allergy, which caused her to experience severe stomach pain and sickness.

As a fellow parent, I'm sure you can imagine that those initial weeks were a testing period for both of us as I navigated the terrain of new motherhood while unravelling the mystery behind my baby's inability to keep down her milk feeds.

The lack of support, coupled with my daughter's allergy, ignited something within me. I was determined to offer the weaning support that was missing and ensure that no other parent felt the same level of anxiety as I did as our weaning journey drew closer.

Crafting recipes to meet Annabelle's dietary needs, without the need to make separate meals for her, became my mission. During Annabelle's nap time, I dedicated moments to jotting down recipe ideas in a small notebook. I'd meticulously test them in the kitchen, making subtle tweaks along the way, and sought feedback from friends and family to refine the flavours. Despite enduring months of severe sleep deprivation and concerns about my return to work, a genuine sense of purpose started to emerge. Nothing brought me greater joy than creating recipes and seeing those I loved, especially Annabelle, enjoy them.

Encouraged by the positive responses to my creations, I took the initiative to educate myself on BLW through courses and books. Eager to share my passion with other parents, in 2015 I started a Facebook page. Almost overnight, the page gained momentum, and I distinctly remember thinking: 'This is my purpose; everything is happening for a reason.' The joy of helping fellow parents and witnessing their little ones relishing my recipes became an unparalleled source of fulfilment.

In the years since the inception of the Facebook page I've developed an array of resources for parents. This includes recipe apps, an educational course and a wealth of support materials designed to guide them through an easy and enjoyable weaning experience.

I find immense joy in devoting my life to supporting fellow parents through my apps and social media platforms. This book extends that commitment, delving even deeper to aid more parents in discovering that weaning can be easy, effortless and fun!

My recipes are uncomplicated and my guidance strives to be simple. My goal is to supply you with everything you need so your baby can grow up enjoying healthy, nutritious and, above all, tasty foods!

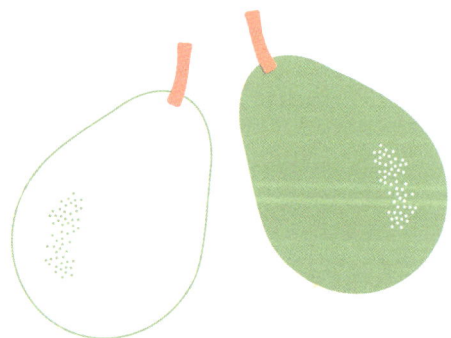

HOW TO USE THIS BOOK

This book has been designed to make baby-led weaning a calm and enjoyable experience for you and your baby.

Most parents' minds begin swirling with questions as this exciting new journey draws closer, and if your own mind feels like a whirlwind, rest assured that by the time you finish reading this book, you will be well equipped and full of confidence to embark on this new adventure.

To make this book easy to digest, it's been divided into three chapters of practical information, followed by a chapter of tips and tricks for the kitchen, and finally the all-important recipes. As you navigate these chapters, consider using sticky tabs or Post-it notes to mark key information for quick reference. With the unpredictability of a baby's needs, I also recommend keeping a bookmark handy so you can pick up where you left off at a moment's notice.

I begin the book by discussing the fundamental principles of BLW, because the more you understand this approach, the more confidence you will have to embrace it and fearlessly work through any hurdles.

Following this, I delve into your baby's nutritional needs, offering guidance on safe foods and foods that should be limited or avoided altogether. I also discuss how to manage specific dietary requirements and the importance of variety. This nutritional chapter, which has been verified by a paediatric dietitian and feeding specialist, leaves no stone unturned and will ensure your baby gets the healthiest start.

We will then transition into the practical logistics of adopting baby-led weaning. In this chapter I provide you with a comprehensive, stress-free guide to getting your BLW journey started, covering various approaches, essential tools and equipment, and expert tips to tackle any challenges you may encounter. I also dedicate some of this chapter to specific topics concerning your baby's safety and safe food preparation practices. Again, rest assured, every detail of this chapter has been meticulously checked and verified by an expert in safe eating practices for babies and children.

Finally, I present a collection of 60 quick-and-easy family recipes, each requiring no more than 20 minutes of your valuable time. I understand the challenges of juggling cooking with the demands of being a busy parent. And too much time spent in the kitchen can make cooking feel like a chore. I want you to enjoy preparing the recipes as much as you do tucking into them with your little one.

In the Rise and Shine chapter (see page 96), you will find some incredibly wholesome recipes packed with nutritious ingredients designed to give you and your family the best start to your day. Breakfast has always been my favourite meal of the day, and I enjoyed taking inspiration from my own childhood when developing this chapter – so if you're a fellow child of the 90s, you may notice some salutes to this vibrant era! I know that, for parents, mornings can be quite a tricky time, so if yours are a mad, crazy dash like mine, then please don't fret; these recipes are easy to prepare in advance and most freeze like a dream, so all you need to do in the morning is enjoy them.

The Yummy Easy-peasy Lunches (see page 120) presented here are intentionally simple and realistically manageable, offering ideas that can become staples in your routine. They also provide a perfect opportunity to repurpose leftovers, encouraging you to get creative with ingredients, so please feel free to add whatever leftover vegetables or meat you have to the recipes.

There are delicious and filing No-fuss Dinners (see page 142) that won't break the bank, with exciting fakeaway options such as curries and burger wraps, defying the notion that weaning meals must be bland and boring.

As you delve into the Tiny Bites and Treats (see page 164) you will uncover an array of finger foods and tasty treats that will complement any meal. Perfect for those on the move, these quick and easy-to-pack options are a game-changer, and a lifesaver for parents who may be navigating the world of childcare. And as the baker, you'll find yourself obliged to indulge in a taste test before sharing the joy!

Time and time again, when I'm asked how to make weaning as easy as possible, I tell parents to batch cook. If you're already cooking, just double or triple the recipe. With this approach, you will always have a handy freezer stash and considerably reduce the time spent cooking. To assist you with this I have added 12 make-ahead Freezer Stash recipes (see page 187).

As an adult, you may find some of these recipes a little bland without any added salt. Therefore, I encourage you to add a little salt or extra spice to your own portion to intensify the flavours and ensure you can enjoy the recipes as much as your little one.

All recipes are suitable for children aged six months and above. Alongside each one I provide guidance on adapting ingredients to meet specific dietary requirements to assist those managing allergies and intolerances.

Important: before you start baby-led weaning, please consult your doctor to ensure this form of weaning is appropriate and safe for your child.

RECIPE ICONS

All recipes are clearly marked with dietary and storage icons.

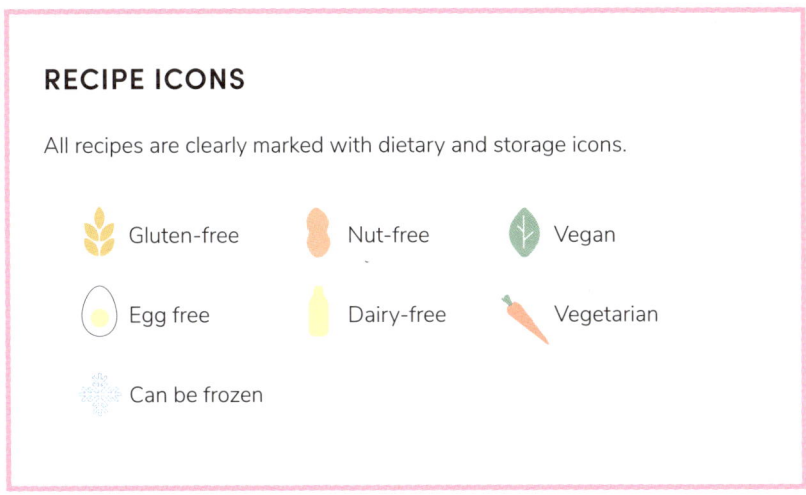

Gluten-free

Nut-free

Vegan

Egg free

Dairy-free

Vegetarian

Can be frozen

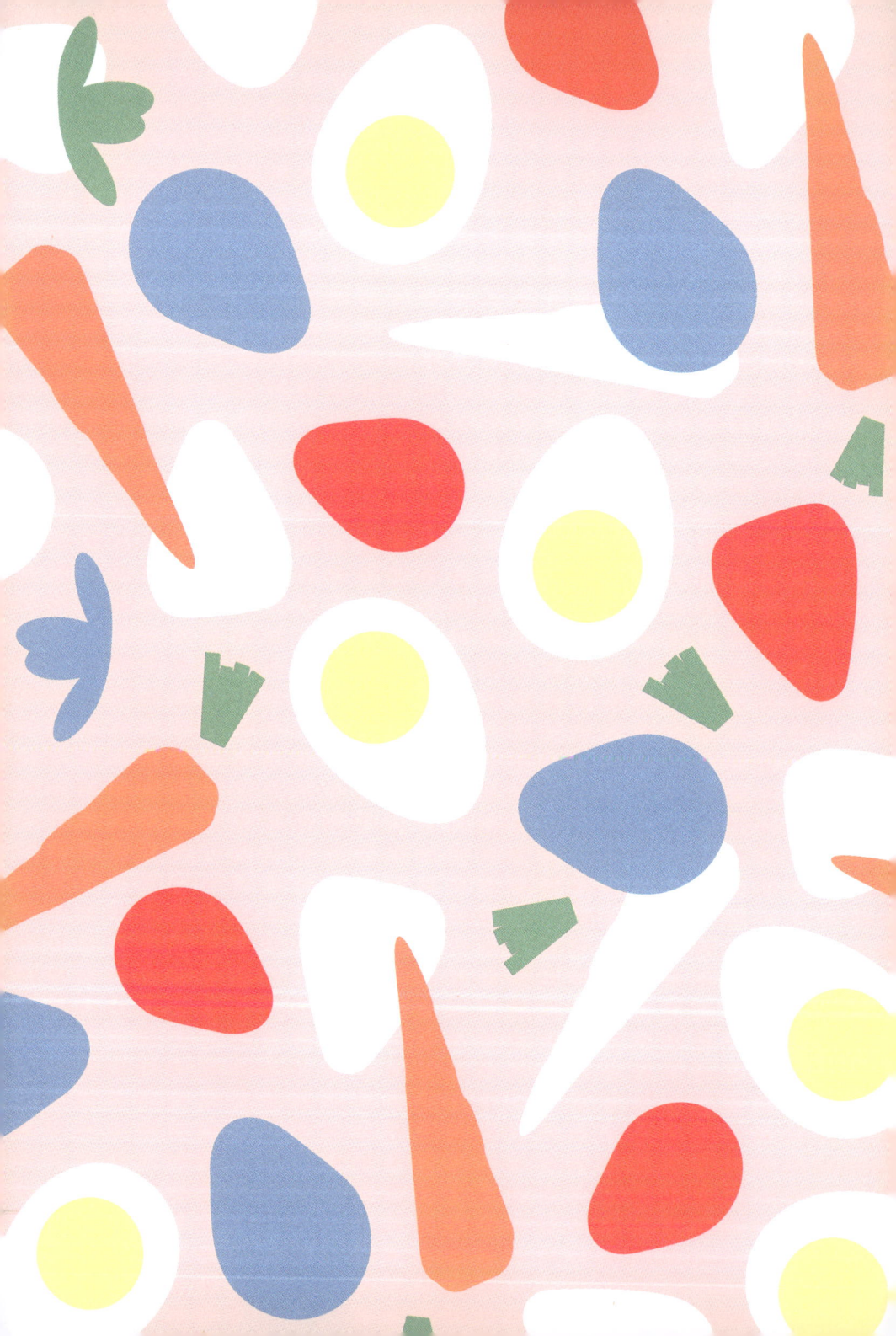

The Basics

In the world of parenting and nutrition, baby-led weaning (BLW) has emerged as a transformative approach to introducing solid foods to infants. It allows little ones to embark on a culinary journey by offering them smaller portions of family meals from the age of six months, opening the door to a world of new experiences.

I am firmly against the notion of 'baby food', as distinct from other foods, and encourage you to quash this preconception, as deeply embedded as it may be. As you will discover in this book, there is very little a baby can't enjoy!

In the following chapter, I'll explore the key advantages of this approach, from promoting independence to nurturing your baby's discovery of tastes and textures, and address the signs of readiness, dispelling common misconceptions and emphasizing the importance of patience in this journey. Above all, I want to highlight the significance of trusting your baby to lead the way, allowing them to explore, learn and develop their relationship with food at their own pace. BLW is not just about feeding; it's about fostering a lifelong love for nutritious and varied foods, one bite at a time.

WHAT IS BABY-LED WEANING?

Baby-led weaning is a weaning approach in which you skip the purée stage of traditional weaning and offer your baby smaller portions of your own meals from six months of age. Unlike the conventional method of spoon-feeding purées, BLW allows babies to take the lead, exploring food and feeding themselves from the very beginning of their weaning journey. This approach empowers infants, enabling them to actively participate in mealtimes, promoting independence and fostering a positive relationship with food from day one. At its core, BLW is about granting infants a say in their journey towards solid foods.

One of the key principles of BLW is that babies are introduced to solid foods when they are developmentally ready, usually around six months of age. At this stage, most babies can sit up unassisted and have developed the necessary motor skills to grasp and bring food to their mouths. Instead of puréeing foods, parents offer soft, appropriately sized pieces of food that babies can pick up, explore and gum on. This not only encourages the development of fine motor skills and hand-eye coordination, but also allows babies to explore a variety of textures, flavours and colours.

Unlike the historical shift towards the early introduction of solids at four months, BLW adheres to the recommendations of the UK's National Health Service (NHS) and the World Health Organization (WHO), advising parents to wait until their babies are developmentally ready for solid food, typically around the six-month mark.

The shift in the age at which babies were introduced to solids reflects a broader trend influenced by societal changes and technological advancements. Until the 1930s, the prevailing practice was to delay introducing solid foods until a baby reached six months. However, the landscape changed significantly with the advent of pre-packaged foods and innovative kitchen appliances, such as the food processor, which streamlined baby food preparation. Consequently, the recommended age for introducing solids dropped to earlier, at four months.

The rationale behind this shift was rooted in the convenience offered by commercial baby food and the ease of processing it into smooth purées. This period marked a departure from the traditional practice of waiting until six months when most babies are developmentally prepared to consume solid foods safely without the need for purées.

Yet while we often associate BLW with contemporary parenting approaches, the concept has historical roots that precede the era of convenience foods and commercially available jars and pouches. Before the widespread availability of these products, parents commonly engaged in a simplified form of BLW. In this approach, babies would be offered small, manageable pieces of their parents' food, introducing solids in a way that aligned with the child's developmental readiness.

The simplicity of this earlier form of BLW highlights the intuitive nature of introducing solid foods to infants. In contrast to the processed purées that gained popularity, this approach emphasized a more natural progression, allowing babies to explore and engage with food in a manner that complemented their developmental milestones. Today, as we reconsider and adapt our own approach to feeding infants, there is a resurgence of interest in the principles of BLW, signalling a return to a more intuitive method of introducing solid foods, one that allows your baby to form positive eating habits that can follow them through childhood and into their adult life.

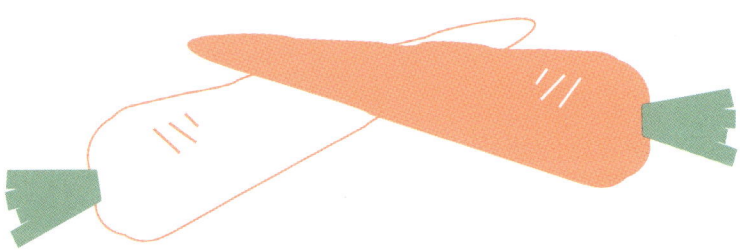

WHAT ARE THE BENEFITS OF BABY-LED WEANING?

» BLW introduces your baby to a broad range of textures and flavours from day one, which can help reduce the risk of picky-eating habits later in life. Many parents attest that babies who independently select their food tend to exhibit more diverse food choices as they develop into childhood.

» BLW empowers your baby to take an active role in their feeding journey, allowing them to grasp and explore food on their own terms, fostering independence. BLW assists in the development and refinement of hand-eye coordination and fine motor skills.

» BLW allows your baby to eat as much as they need in their own time, setting the foundations for healthy eating habits. It also encourages babies to listen to their hunger and fullness cues, helping children to understand when they need to eat, and when they should stop.

» BLW means that your baby can be offered the same food as the rest of the family without additional preparation. This can help to save time and money by eliminating the need to cook separate meals for your baby.

» Baby-led weaning can make mealtime a more inclusive and enjoyable family experience, as babies enjoy the same meals as the rest of the family, facilitating social interaction, bonding and an opportunity to work on their communication skills.

COMMON BABY-LED WEANING MYTHS

MYTH 1:
BLW IS ONLY FOR BABIES WITH TEETH
Reality: BLW is designed to accommodate babies who are just beginning to explore solid foods. Even without teeth, babies can use their strong gums to chew soft, age-appropriate foods. The approach focuses on developing oral motor skills, allowing babies to explore and learn to manipulate various textures.

MYTH 2: BLW MEANS GIVING UP CONTROL OF HOW MUCH YOUR BABY EATS

Reality: While BLW encourages independence, it doesn't mean parents lose control. Parents still play a crucial role in selecting appropriate foods, ensuring a safe eating environment and monitoring their baby's progress. It's a collaborative approach that empowers babies to self-feed within a guided framework.

MYTH 3: BABIES WILL NOT GET ENOUGH IRON

Reality: With considered food choices, babies can receive sufficient iron through BLW. Iron-rich foods such as meat, beans and iron-fortified cereals can all be introduced, encouraging a diverse diet and supporting overall nutritional intake. See pages 28–29 for more on nutrition.

MYTH 4: BLW TAKES LONGER THAN TRADITIONAL WEANING

Reality: BLW can be very time-efficient. While it may take a little longer for babies to master self-feeding, it eliminates the need for preparing separate purées. And as babies become more adept at feeding themselves, the process becomes quicker, with less time spent helping with spoon-feeding.

MYTH 5: BLW INCREASES THE RISK OF CHOKING

Reality: When foods are prepared correctly, following the correct advice and support about feeding and food preparation, BLW does not increase the risk of choking. See pages 58–59 for more information.

MYTH 6: BABIES WILL NOT GAIN ENOUGH WEIGHT WITH BLW

Reality: Throughout the initial six months of weaning, breast or formula milk remains crucial for meeting your baby's essential caloric and nutritional requirements. A 2017 study investigating behaviours linked to the BLW method, its results and potential influencing factors revealed that a substantial majority of infants following both baby-led and traditional weaning approaches maintained a healthy weight. The study reported that 'The majority of children exhibited a healthy weight (81 per cent for BLW and 84 per cent for traditional weaning)'.

MYTH 7: BLW ONLY WORKS FOR CERTAIN TYPES OF FAMILIES

Reality: BLW is adaptable to various family dynamics and lifestyles. Families with diverse cultural backgrounds, dietary preferences and schedules can implement it. The principle of allowing babies to self-feed and explore food applies universally.

READINESS

As mentioned, the UK's National Health Service (NHS) and the World Health Organization (WHO) recommend waiting until your baby is around six months old before offering solids. Observing a baby's unique developmental readiness for introducing solids safely is crucial – each infant will be prepared to commence this transition at their own pace.

Starting solids before your baby is developmentally ready can put them at greater risk of choking. Therefore, it's essential you can tick off *all* the readiness signs in the chart below before you begin. Once all the boxes in the chart are ticked, you can be assured your baby is ready to start their weaning journey safely.

Readiness signs:
» Your baby can sit up with little or no support
» Your baby can hold their head steady
» Your baby can successfully reach out, grab and bring toys to their mouth
» Your baby's tongue thrust reflex is diminishing

WHAT IS THE TONGUE TRUST REFLEX?

Also known as the extrusion reflex, this is an automatic response in infants in which the tongue protrudes outwards when the lips are touched or when a foreign object is placed in the mouth, helping in breastfeeding and early feeding behaviours. As a child matures, this reflex diminishes (usually around four to six months), allowing for more coordinated and controlled tongue movements during eating and speech development.

Signs that are sometimes confused for readiness:

1. **Your baby is picking up objects and putting them in their mouth**. Babies naturally put everything in their mouths. This is how they learn and discover the world around them. This action alone is not a sign of readiness to start solids.
2. **Your baby is not sleeping through the night**. It's normal for a baby to not sleep through, and it doesn't indicate a readiness for solids.
3. **Your baby wants extra milk feeds.** Again, this is normal and not a sign of readiness.

Remember, there is no rush.

Understandably, parents are often worried about weaning. Please try to put any fears aside at the start of your journey because if you are anxious or stressed, your baby will pick up on it. The most important thing when you start weaning is to get your baby used to trying lots of different tastes and textures. A tense atmosphere can leave your little one feeling stressed and unwilling to participate in mealtimes with eagerness and confidence. Instead, they might display caution and show cues such as fussiness, signalling that the mealtime is over and they want to be removed from the stressful environment. Take it slow and easy.

In the first few weeks, your baby will start to learn how to move food around their mouth and swallow it. Until your baby starts to master these key skills, it's likely that lots of food will be pushed or spat out. This is normal. Weaning is a marathon, not a sprint, and is about so much more than just the food itself. Please be assured that most of your baby's nutritional needs will still be met from breast or formula milk at this stage, and for the first couple of months of weaning, the amount of food they consume is not important. Slow and steady progress is key.

From my personal experience, Annabelle was about nine months old when she started to get to grips with self-feeding, while my twin boys got the hang of it earlier, at around seven months. I put this down to two things: one, every baby is different; and two, the twins ate their meals with their big sister, whom they love and adore, and mimicking her encouraged them considerably.

Baby-led weaning is exactly that: baby-led. The philosophy is to trust in your baby and let them lead the way so that they can explore at their own pace, allowing them to develop in their own time and learn to regulate their own appetite. Some babies take a keen interest in food immediately, while others can take a good couple of months to show an interest. Much like every other milestone – smiling, walking, talking – you find that all babies catch up with each other eventually. Worrying will not benefit you or your baby, but I do appreciate that this can be easier said than done at times.

REDUCING MILK INTAKE

As you and your baby navigate the world of BLW from six to twelve months, another significant aspect of their development unfolds: the gradual transition from milk feeds to a more diversified and solid-based diet. Around six months, as your baby begins to explore the exciting realm of solids, they gradually reduce their reliance on milk feeds. One fundamental tenet of BLW is to trust your baby's cues. As they become more proficient eaters, they may naturally show less interest in milk feeds.

Trust your baby to lead the way. They'll explore in their own time, in their own way and at their own pace.

BALANCING SOLIDS AND MILK

While introducing solids, it's crucial to maintain a balance between milk and solid feeds. Breast milk or formula remains the primary source of nutrition during this period, providing essential nutrients and ensuring your baby's overall growth and development. Here are some key things to keep in mind:

PROGRESSIVE CHANGES: ADAPTING TO BABY'S PACE

Between six and twelve months, you may notice a gradual decrease in the frequency and volume of milk feeds. This transition is a natural part of your baby's development and their growing ability to derive nourishment from a diverse range of solid foods.

MEALTIME ROUTINES: ESTABLISHING HEALTHY HABITS

Establishing regular mealtimes helps to create a structured routine for your baby. Offer solids before milk feeds to encourage them to explore and enjoy a variety of foods. This approach fosters a positive relationship with food, allowing your baby to savour the sensory experience of eating.

NHS advice states that breast milk or first infant formula should be their main drink during the first year. You can continue breastfeeding for as long as you both want. Remember your baby's tummy is tiny and fills up quickly, so offer milk feeds after solids.

INDIVIDUAL VARIATIONS: EVERY BABY IS UNIQUE

It's essential to recognize that every baby follows their own timeline. Some may adapt quickly to a more solid-focused diet, while others will prefer a gradual transition. Pay attention to your baby's signals, be flexible, and consult your GP if you have concerns about their nutritional intake.

NUTRITIONAL CONSIDERATIONS: ENSURING ADEQUATE NUTRITION

As milk feeds decrease, focus on offering nutrient-dense foods to meet your baby's growing nutritional needs. Include a variety of fruits, vegetables, proteins, fats and grains to ensure a balanced diet. Offer water during mealtimes to keep your baby hydrated.

CELEBRATING MILESTONES: EMBRACING INDEPENDENCE

Dropping milk feeds signifies a significant milestone in your baby's journey towards independence. These moments are not only about nutrition, but also about fostering a positive attitude towards eating.

GETTING OTHERS ON BOARD WITH BABY-LED WEANING

I am a big advocate of baby-led weaning. However, I fully appreciate that not everyone believes in this method of weaning, at least initially. For older carers, spoon-feeding is likely the primary method that they are familiar and feel confident with, as it's probably the approach they took with their own children. BLW will feel like a new and perhaps even 'experimental' method of weaning, and there may be a period of adjustment while they get to grips with the concept.

High childcare costs mean grandparents are increasingly helping out with the care of their grandchildren, so it's essential they support your weaning choices. Fortunately, most are open to new approaches and understand that things change over the years, but for some it's a step too far, and fears of choking or messy meals understandably cause stress and anxiety.

I have encountered parents who are nervous about returning to work because grandparents will be helping with childcare but will not support their choice of BLW. If you are concerned about this, I would like to offer some tips for overcoming this challenge and getting them fully on board. But before I do, I must mention that most grandparents and older caregivers who have felt unsure about BLW have, in my experience, eventually come around to the approach when they witness its wonders first-hand – they've even been known to rave about it to everyone and anyone who will listen!

1. DO SOME TRIAL RUNS

Before leaving your baby for the first time, I recommend inviting grandparents or carers over to eat a few meals with you and your baby, to get in some low-pressure BLW trial runs. This can help them to get comfortable with the process and hopefully see that it's not so daunting after all.

These shared mealtimes are a good opportunity to educate. I recommend discussing the food you've selected, how you prepared it and why. Ask them if they have any questions, and answer them without showing frustration, even if they seem trivial. Remember, this is all brand new to them.

This is a good chance for them to see what to do if your baby gags, without the pressure of being the one 'in charge'. Hopefully, they will begin to understand how fantastic it is when they experience the reality of BLW, or at least start coming around to the idea.

2. PREPARE FOODS INITIALLY

To take the pressure off initially, I recommend you prepare meals yourself in advance. This removes the stress of grandparents or carers having to prepare and cook the food safely, as it's already been done for them. As well as giving you some control and peace of mind over what is being served, it also allows grandparents to learn

about what you are offering, so they can build their own knowledge and understanding of best practices.

At drop-off, you can briefly discuss your food choices and explain your reasoning. Even though you may be confident your little one can go to town on a steak, maybe start off with some steamed or roasted veggies until the carer builds their confidence.

3. MEAL PLAN ENTRY-LEVEL 'SAFE' FOODS

You may decide you want to continue preparing your baby's meals long-term; however, if you would like to give your carers more control and yourself one less thing to do, you could suggest a weekly meal plan of more basic foods until they are feeling more confident. This way, you will still have control and know what your baby is eating, and it will allow them some time to prepare the food in advance.

4. EDUCATE

Consider offering grandparents and carers a copy of this book. In doing so, they can learn about all the wonderful benefits of BLW and have 60 easy recipes in their arsenal. My baby-led weaning course is also available, which can be watched and referred back to as much as needed (see page 204). Perhaps you could watch together initially, discussing the topics after each chapter.

Nutrition and Safety

Good nutrition is paramount in the remarkable journey of a baby's first year, characterized by exponential growth and development. Witnessing your baby's weight doubling by six months and tripling by 12 months demonstrates the critical role of nutrition in shaping their physical, cognitive and emotional well-being.

This chapter looks at the essential nutrients that form the foundation of a baby's diet, and unfolds the intricacies of meeting your baby's nutritional requirements, ensuring a seamless transition from exclusive milk feeds to a rich, diverse diet supporting optimal growth. Each element contributes uniquely to their development, from energy to proteins, carbohydrates to fats, and a spectrum of vital vitamins and minerals. I explore the dynamic interplay of these nutritional components, emphasizing the evolving needs of infants as they progress from the delicate stage of newborn to the robust explorer of their environment at 12 months.

As you embark on your baby-led weaning (BLW) journey, ensuring the safety and well-being of your little one is paramount. This chapter will equip you with the knowledge and skills necessary to minimize risks and ensure a smooth transition to solid foods. In the latter part of the chapter I will discuss the essential aspects of safety, exploring the crucial distinction between choking and gagging, and giving you the confidence to navigate these situations calmly and effectively. I will also guide you through the importance of appropriately preparing and serving foods to reduce choking risks. Learning to cut, cook and introduce various foods safely is key to a successful BLW experience.

NUTRITIONAL REQUIREMENTS FOR INFANTS

During the crucial first year of a baby's life, as infants gain weight and start to explore the world around them, absorbing a great number sensory experiences, the role of nutrition becomes even more pronounced, not only to fuel their growing bodies but as a foundational component in shaping their lifelong health and well-being.

BABY'S ESSENTIAL NUTRIENTS

» **Energy (calories):** Infants require substantial energy for growth, activity and metabolic processes. Caloric needs vary depending on factors such as age, weight and activity level, but on average, the requirements fall between 72 and 96 kcal/kg/day between six and 12 months.

» **Protein:** Protein is essential for the growth and development of muscles, organs and tissues. Some foods high in protein include eggs, nuts, meat, cottage cheese, yoghurt and lentils.

» **Carbohydrates:** Carbohydrates are the primary source of energy for infants. As a guideline, about 40–50 per cent of an infant's total daily calories should come from carbohydrates. Nourishing carbohydrates – such as grains, vegetables, fruits and beans – are rich sources of vitamins, minerals and fibre, promoting overall health and well-being.

» **Fats**: Fats are crucial for brain development, as well as the absorption of fat-soluble vitamins (A, D, E and K). Healthy fats include avocados, olive oil, nuts and oily fish, contributing essential nutrients like omega-3 fatty acids. These fats support heart health, aid in nutrient absorption and provide sustained energy, forming a crucial part of a balanced and nutritious diet.

» **Vitamins:** Vitamins play a vital role in various metabolic processes. Key infant vitamins include vitamin D for bone and immune health, vitamin K for blood clotting and vitamin C for immune health, overall growth and development.

» **Minerals**: Essential minerals for infants include calcium, phosphorus, iron and zinc. Calcium and phosphorus are vital for bone development, iron is necessary for healthy blood and zinc supports growth and immune function.

» **Water:** Infants have a higher percentage of water in their bodies than adults and can become dehydrated more quickly due to their underdeveloped fluid-regulating system, elevated body-water content, increased metabolic rate and limited thirst response. Water can be introduced in a sippy cup or small open cup, with meals, from the age of six months to encourage healthy drinking habits and help to support the skills needed to drink from a cup.

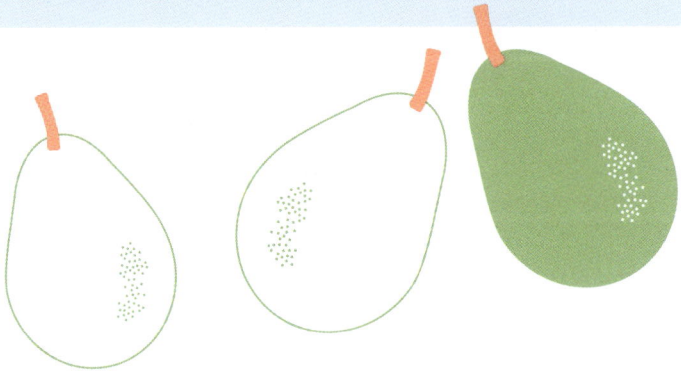

MEETING NUTRITIONAL REQUIREMENTS

From birth until six months, breast and/or formula milk will meet your baby's unique nutritional requirements. From six months of age onwards, it will continue to contribute to their requirements alongside the introduction of complementary foods. Of course, just because your baby reaches 12 months, you don't need to completely cut off milk feeds; continue to offer milk for as long as you wish, alongside solid foods. By offering a variety of nutrition-dense foods from day one of your baby's weaning journey, you will encourage a diet full of goodness to support their optimal health.

HOW MUCH SHOULD MY BABY BE EATING?

The question of how much a baby should eat is a common concern for parents venturing into BLW. There's no one-size-fits-all answer, however; it's all about your baby and their distinctive needs and preferences.

Babies are fascinatingly unique in their eating habits. Some seem to have an insatiable appetite, leaving you in awe and wondering where all that food could go. On the flip side, others find contentment in smaller portions, and that's perfectly okay. I've witnessed six-month-olds out-eat their ten-month-old counterparts – a testament to the individuality of each little one's journey.

Baby-led weaning, in its essence, celebrates this individuality. One of the remarkable aspects of BLW as a parent is relinquishing control over how much your baby eats. Instead, we entrust this to their innate ability to self-regulate – a skill that babies excel at, barring any medical conditions. The likelihood of a baby not eating enough when offered a healthy, balanced diet that caters to their nutritional needs is very low.

It's crucial to acknowledge that, in the same way as adults, babies have days when hunger strikes more fiercely than others. Their growth rate also naturally slows as they pass 12 months, impacting their appetite accordingly. This variance is not only normal but expected. Of course, we also have to take into consideration that teething and illness can impact your baby's desire to eat.

It's easy to compare your baby's eating habits with others (I know I have!), triggering concerns about whether they're consuming too much or too little. Yet, the beauty of a baby's instinctive self-regulation should provide solace. Your baby knows how much they need to thrive.

As you embark on this journey of BLW, embrace your baby's individual, unique appetite. Trust their cues, celebrate their individuality and rest assured that babies are proficient at knowing what's right for them.

HOW MUCH SHOULD I PLATE UP?

It's easy to forget sometimes that babies' tummies are tiny and don't need significant portions of food. Keeping portions small can prevent your baby from feeling overwhelmed by the quantity of food in front of them and will help to avoid food waste. Feel free to add more to your baby's plate as necessary, but starting with a smaller portion is a wise strategy for avoiding overwhelm.

THE IMPORTANCE OF VARIETY

I'm often asked what is the most important advice I can give to parents before they start BLW. And the answer is simple: offer as much variety as possible before your baby's first birthday. This single tip can significantly impact your infant's eating habits in the long term, reducing your mental load, stress levels and time spent preparing meals.

Baby-led weaning is a journey of discovery that allows babies to experience a diverse range of foods in their first year of life. By offering a wide variety, you can encourage positive eating habits and promote the development of a healthy, well-rounded palate.

FAMILIAR FOODS

Most babies will eat anything; they are growing rapidly and enjoy trying any tasty creation. However, toddlers can be more of a challenge, and often gravitate towards familiar foods.

For toddlers, familiarity provides a sense of comfort and security. They are at an age where they are developing independence and testing boundaries, so the familiar can be a reassuring constant in their rapidly changing world. Familiar foods are like old friends: they offer a predictable taste and texture that toddlers can trust, reducing the uncertainty that can accompany trying new foods.

Toddlers are naturally curious, but can be wary of the unknown. They are more likely to accept foods they have already seen, smelled and tasted. The phenomenon known as 'food neophobia' is a common developmental stage in early childhood. Food neophobia is a hesitancy to consume or a tendency to avoid unfamiliar foods. Therefore, toddlers may hesitate to try new foods, even if they look enticing, as they are hardwired to be cautious of potential threats. Consequently, they often stick to what they know, favouring foods that have been part of their dietary repertoire since infancy and which are therefore more predictable.

By offering lots of variety between the ages of six to twelve months, you can create an arsenal of familiar foods your baby is happy to continue enjoying as they move into their toddler years.

AVOID 'BABY AND TODDLER FOOD'

The food industry has developed a range of foods – including jars, frozen meals and snacks – designed specifically for babies and toddlers. While these foods might look fun, light-hearted and healthy, this is usually down to the packaging and clever marketing strategies; in most instances, these foods can still contain added sugars (e.g. as fruit concentrates), salt and highly processed ingredients.

If you want to know whether a product is healthy for your family, one way to tell is to look at the ingredients it contains. If it has a long list of ingredients that you don't recognize, which look like they belong on a scientific chart rather than an ingredients list, you may want to consider limiting or reducing consumption of them. I'm not advocating cutting these foods out entirely, though. I know full well the juggle of parenthood, and at times we need to lean on convenience foods for our own mental health and well-being.

I do, however, encourage parents to dismiss the notion of 'baby and toddler foods' and see food as a whole for everyone, regardless of age. It's easy to get into the habit of relying on speedy convenience foods, and in moderation (for our sanity!) they are fine, but try not to lean on them too heavily as it will do you no favours in the long run. There is very little a baby cannot eat, and offering meals eaten by the whole family will prevent your baby from becoming accustomed to these pre-packed baby and toddler foods.

The aim is to avoid your baby expecting food to look or taste a certain (bland) way – we want them to develop a love of flavour and to enjoy a broad spectrum of tastes and textures.

DIVERSE NUTRITION

Offering a wide array of foods is essential for providing infants with the full range of nutritional requirements. Different foods contain different vitamins, minerals and essential nutrients, and by introducing a variety of fruits, vegetables, proteins, fats and grains, you can ensure that your baby receives a balanced diet. This diversity supports optimal growth and development during this crucial stage of life.

Meals don't need to be complicated; they just need to be varied. I often lean on jacket potatoes, frozen vegetables, tinned tuna and baked beans for easy mid-week meals to fit between school and nursery pick-ups and after-school clubs; simple meals can be just as diverse as more complex ones. It's also important to let go of your own preferences, and if you're fussy with certain foods, to push yourself to try them again, perhaps in a new way you might enjoy more.

It has been shown that repeated exposure to foods or drinks you dislike can often result in you actually liking them. This idea is supported by Guy Crosby, Adjunct Associate Professor of Nutrition at Harvard University's T.H. Chan School of Public Health, who explains; 'It is possible to learn to like tastes that a person finds unpleasant.'

To explore this concept further, I conducted a week-long experiment with the help of my husband and a very supportive friend. During this time, I opted to enjoy my morning coffee without the habitual teaspoon of sugar. Simultaneously, my husband, Steve, who traditionally despises peanut butter, agreed to have it on toast for breakfast. Additionally, a friend, known for disdainfully referring to fruit teas as 'dishwater liquid', committed to sipping one every night before bedtime.

Remarkably, after just four days, we all discovered that our initial aversions had notably softened, and by the end of the week, we had actually developed a genuine fondness for them!

Please give this a try and see for yourself. Ultimately, our children's eating habits will mimic our own, so setting a good example is paramount.

ENJOYMENT

Mealtimes should be an enjoyable and positive experience. Providing an array of colourful, flavourful and textured foods can make mealtimes more exciting for babies, captivating their interest and enthusiasm for eating and creating positive associations. You can also have fun serving foods differently, with crinkle and cookie cutters for example, so it never gets boring.

FOOD REFUSAL

Babies and toddlers may refuse food for various reasons and this behaviour is a normal part of their development. Some common reasons include:

» **Developmental stage:** Toddlers are still developing their taste preferences and may naturally exhibit caution or reluctance to try new foods.

» **Sensory sensitivities:** Heightened sensitivity to textures, smells or tastes can make toddlers selective in their food choices.

» **Autonomy and control:** Seeking independence, toddlers may assert control over their environment, including their food choices, as a way of expressing autonomy.

» **Exploration and experimentation:** Toddlers explore their world through experimentation, including trying different foods. Rejecting certain foods can be part of this learning process.

» **Preference for familiarity:** Toddlers often prefer familiar foods, and any deviation from the familiar may be met with resistance. This preference is a normal aspect of their development.

» **Parental influence:** Toddlers may mimic the attitudes and preferences of parents or caregivers, and adverse reactions to certain foods can influence their choices.

» **Temporary aversions:** Toddlers may experience temporary aversions due to illness or teething, affecting their appetite and willingness to eat (see page 36).

» **Communication challenges:** Toddlers may need help verbally expressing their likes or dislikes, leading to food refusal to communicate their preferences.

It's essential to approach toddler feeding with patience, provide a variety of nutritious foods and create positive mealtime environments. Gradual exposure to new foods and involving toddlers in meal preparation can encourage a diverse and healthy diet over time. I talk in more depth about food refusal and tools you can use to over this behaviour on page 78.

ILLNESS, BAD HABITS AND MINDSET

When your baby or toddler becomes unwell, it can be a gruelling time for parents, and we naturally want to help our little ones and take away their suffering. The worst three days of my parenting journey so far (aside from the newborn vomit fest) was when Annabelle got chickenpox. I tried everything, but she was in a constant state of distress, and I honestly wanted the ground to swallow me whole.

If your infant is unwell and refusing to eat, I do not recommend you encourage them to eat by tempting them with their favourite foods. By offering alternative foods after initial refusal, we demonstrate that they will get their favourites if other food is not eaten. This can be especially risky with toddlers striving for control. They will soon realize that refusing to eat is an easy way to control the food on their plate and can start limiting the variety of foods they accept.

Therefore, it's important that even through illness you keep a strong mindset and do not alter your feeding habits; continue to offer a variety of meals as usual, both favourites and non-favourites. Although it's hard, don't worry if food goes uneaten. This is not picky eating. This is your child feeling unwell and being off their food like any adult. By offering varied meals as usual – which can of course *include* their most loved foods – you can ensure your baby or toddler will resume their everyday eating habits once they feel better.

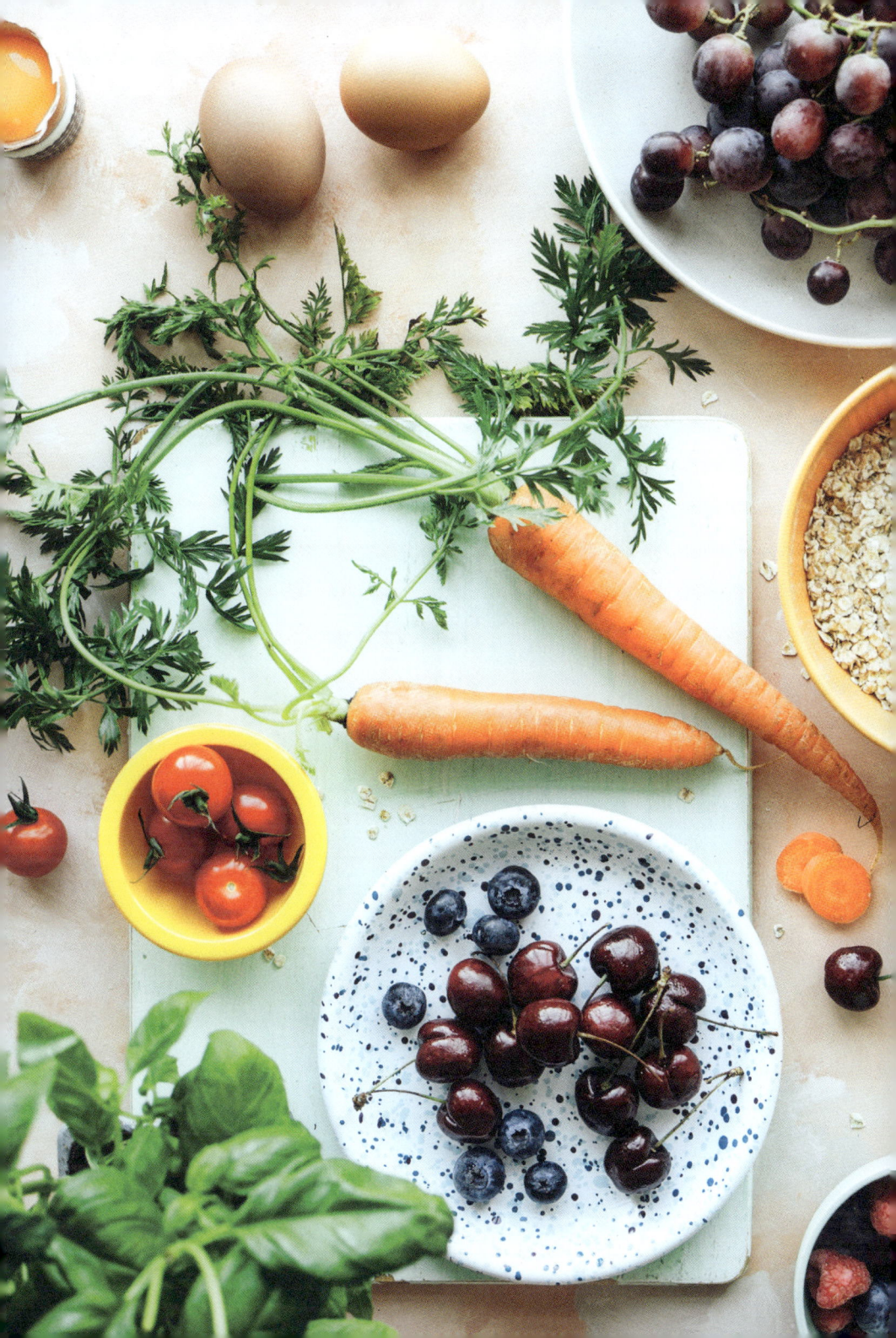

FIRST FOOD CHECKLIST FOR BABY-LED WEANING

VEGETABLES

- Artichoke
- Asparagus
- Aubergine (eggplant)
- Beetroot (beets)
- Broccoli
- Brussels sprouts
- Butternut squash
- Cabbage
- Carrot
- Cauliflower
- Celeriac (celery root)
- Courgette (zucchini)
- Cucumber
- Garlic
- Ginger
- Green beans
- Kale
- Leek
- Lettuce
- Mushrooms
- Onion
- Parsnip
- Peas
- Pepper
- Potato
- Pumpkin
- Rhubarb
- Spinach
- Swede (rutabaga)
- Sweetcorn
- Sweet potato

FRUITS

- Apple
- Apricot
- Avocado
- Banana
- Blackberry
- Blackcurrant
- Blueberry
- Cherry
- Coconut
- Cranberry
- Grape
- Grapefruit
- Kiwi
- Lemon
- Lime
- Mango
- Melon
- Nectarine
- Orange
- Passion fruit
- Peach
- Pear
- Pineapple
- Plum
- Prune
- Raspberry
- Strawberry
- Tangerine
- Tomato
- Watermelon

BEANS & LEGUMES

- Black beans
- Cannellini (white) beans
- Chickpeas (garbanzos)
- Edamame beans
- Lentils
- Peas
- Peanut*
- Pinto beans
- Kidney beans
- Tofu

NUTS & SEEDS*

- Almond
- Cashew
- Chia seeds
- Hazelnut
- Pecan
- Pistachio
- Tahini
- Walnut

MEAT

- Beef
- Chicken
- Chicken liver
- Lamb
- Pork
- Turkey

SEAFOOD

- Bass
- Cod
- Crab
- Halibut
- Herring
- Prawn (shrimp)
- Salmon
- Sardine
- Trout
- Tuna

GRAINS

- Bread
- Couscous
- Egg noodles
- Oats
- Pasta
- Quinoa
- White rice
- Brown rice
- Any other options e.g. barley, buckwheat, etc.

DAIRY & EGGS

- Cow's milk
- Custard
- Hard cheese e.g. Cheddar, Gruyère, Emmental
- Soft cheese e.g. goat's cheese, mascarpone, mozzarella, ricotta
- Yoghurt
- Eggs

* Nuts and peanuts are a choking hazard; please serve finely diced or ground into butter form.

FOODS TO BE MINDFUL OF OR AVOID

Certain foods pose potential risks to babies or should be used in moderation. Below, I have outlined what to steer clear of and what to exercise caution with when preparing foods for your baby.

SALT

Until they are 12 months old, limit your baby's salt intake to under 1g per day; this can be doubled to 2g from one to three years old. As acknowledged by the NHS, too much salt can be dangerous to your baby's kidney health, so avoid adding salt to their meals, use low-salt options, and limit foods that are high in salt, such as:

» Bacon
» Sausages
» Salted chips
» Crackers
» Crisps
» Pre-packaged meals and takeaways

SUGAR

In its natural forms, such as those found in fruits and some dairy products, sugar is an integral part of a healthy diet, contributing essential energy for a baby's rapid growth and development. However, not all sources of sugar are equal, and moderation remains an essential principle.

Rather than demonizing sugar outright, it's helpful to foster an understanding of the distinction between naturally occurring sugars and added sugars. Natural sugars come packaged with vital nutrients and fibre, enhancing the food's overall nutritional value. Hence, incorporating these sources into a baby's diet is acceptable and often beneficial.

Sugary confectionery and sweetened fruit juices, on the other hand, are examples of sources of added sugars without the accompanying nutritional benefits. Excessive intake can lead to adverse effects, such as an increased risk of tooth decay, which is particularly relevant for infants.

Therefore, while I do not advocate for restricting sugar completely, an approach centred on moderation and informed decision-making is essential.

HONEY

Avoid giving your child honey until they are past 12 months. Honey may contain bacteria that produce toxins harmful to a baby's intestines, leading to a severe condition called infant botulism. If a recipe calls for honey, it can be safely swapped for fruit purée.

WHOLE NUTS AND PEANUTS

Whole nuts and peanuts are a choking risk for children aged five and under. However, it is safe to introduce crushed, ground, smooth nut butter or peanut butter from six months.

CHERRY TOMATOES, OLIVES, POPCORN and OTHER CHOKING HAZARDS

Cherry tomatoes, plum tomatoes, large blueberries, olives and any other foods of a similar shape and size are a choking risk and should be cut into quarters to be made safe.

Popcorn also poses a choking risk, as its flakes and sharp edges have the potential to become lodged in a child's throat, leading to gagging or choking. See page 58 for more on choking.

CHEESES

Cheese provides babies with important nutrients, such as calcium, protein and vitamins. At six months, infants can safely enjoy pasteurized full-fat cheese varieties, including mild Cheddar, cottage cheese and cream cheese.

However, mould-ripened soft cheeses, including Brie, Camembert, goat's milk cheese and blue-veined varieties, pose a potential risk to infants. The concern primarily revolves around the presence of listeria, a harmful bacteria that can lead to listeriosis, a serious infection. Due to their developing immune systems, infants are more susceptible to infections than adults.

Listeria can thrive in the moist environment of mould-ripened soft cheeses, and the consequences of infection can be severe for infants, including symptoms such as fever, irritability and difficulty feeding. Therefore, it is imperative for caregivers to exercise caution and exclude these specific cheeses from an infant's diet during their first year.

It is possible, however, to cook with these cheeses, as the cooking process eliminates the threat of listeria.

EGGS

Eggs can be introduced to a baby's diet at six months of age. They are a nutrient powerhouse, rich in choline, which supports brain function, and high-quality protein, which aids muscle development, and a source of other vitamins and minerals essential to a baby's growth.

The inclusion of raw eggs in a baby's diet poses a potential health risk, primarily due to the fact that they may contain the Salmonella bacteria, which can cause foodborne illness, especially in vulnerable infants with developing immune systems. A Salmonella infection can lead to symptoms such as diarrhoea, vomiting, abdominal cramps and fever, so when introducing eggs to a baby's diet, it is crucial to cook them well to destroy any harmful bacteria.

If you are UK-based, please stick to hens' eggs and look for the 'red lion' stamp on the eggshell or the 'British Lion Quality' label on the egg box. These signify that the eggs have passed rigorous safety standards, making them suitable for consumption in raw or lightly cooked forms from six months of age.

RICE DRINKS

For children under the age of five, it's recommended to refrain from using rice drinks as an alternative to breast milk, infant formula or cow's milk, primarily due to the naturally occurring levels of arsenic it contains.

Although arsenic is naturally found in the environment, rice products tend to absorb higher levels of this element. However, it's important to note that this doesn't necessitate a complete avoidance of rice; regulatory measures are in place to establish acceptable limits for arsenic in food products.

SHELLFISH

Babies should avoid consuming raw or minimally cooked shellfish, such as mussels, clams and oysters, as they increase the risk of food poisoning.

MERCURY-RICH FISH

Avoid giving your baby shark, swordfish or marlin, as these fish contain high levels of mercury that could affect the development of their nervous system.

ALLERGY AND INTOLERANCE AWARENESS

It's important to say that I am not a doctor, so this chapter should not be used in place of any medical advice or diagnosis. I can, however, provide you with well-researched and informed information about allergies and weaning to help you make an informed choice.

What I also have available to share is the lived experience of weaning a baby with a cow's milk protein allergy (CMPA), a personal and, at times, challenging experience.

Annabelle entered the world after an uncomplicated pregnancy and fast birth. At first, it all felt a bit too easy, but little did I know what was to come. The initial ease and newborn bubble soon transformed into a highly challenging period when, after transitioning from breastfeeding to formula, Annabelle began experiencing distressing symptoms – projectile vomiting after every feed, limited restless sleep and evident discomfort in the form of constant grunting and groaning – that left me a shell of my former confident self.

Navigating the uncertainties of early motherhood, I researched and suspected reflux, a condition my mother mentioned mirrored my own infancy. Yet Annabelle's condition persisted, despite trying various remedies like Infacol, gripe water and specialized reflux and comfort formula milk. After two weeks of Annabelle projectile vomiting uncontrollably after every milk feed, I decided I needed to seek help.

Desperate for a solution and not getting any answers from our GP, we sought a paediatrician, opting for a private consultation due to the urgency. Diagnosing reflux, the paediatrician provided medication that offered temporary relief. However, as Annabelle's symptoms resurfaced, an NHS referral finally came through. The new NHS paediatrician believed that Annabelle likely suffered from CMPA, which was the underlying cause of the reflux and constant pain.

Transitioning to a unique formula with the cow's milk protein broken down marked a turning point, alleviating Annabelle's discomfort almost overnight. And as we embarked on the weaning journey, omitting cow's milk became a manageable aspect of our routine. Cooking from scratch ensured control over ingredients, allowing for healthy substitutes and a safe diet, free from cow's milk.

At 13 months, Annabelle slowly and successfully started to manage cow's milk in her diet, leading to her discharge from paediatric care at 14 months. Reflecting on this challenging yet transformative journey, I share our experience to reassure others facing similar hurdles. Managing a baby with a cow's milk allergy is undeniably demanding, but with support, informed choices, and substitutes readily available in today's market, both parent and child can navigate the complexities of dietary restrictions while still enjoying a delicious and varied range of meals.

If you too are managing allergies, you are not alone.

COMMON ALLERGIES

Allergy UK state that 'In the UK, 40% of children have been diagnosed with an allergy. The four most common allergic conditions in children are food allergy, eczema, asthma and hay fever. Allergy symptoms can affect all aspects of a child's day to day life, including their health and well-being, education and social activities. However, with a little watchfulness on the part of parents, and culinary curiosity on the part of infants, most tots can devour their way through this journey with some simple adaptions.

The list below includes the 14 most common food allergies in the UK as defined by Allergy UK. While this list is not exhaustive, it will give you a good idea of which foods to watch out for.

» Celery
» Cereals containing gluten
» Crustaceans
» Eggs
» Fish
» Lupin (a legume belonging to the same plant family as peanuts)
» Milk
» Molluscs

- » Mustard
- » Tree nuts
- » Peanuts
- » Sesame seeds

- » Soya
- » Sulphur dioxide (a preservative found in dried fruits, pickled vegetables, sausages, fruit and vegetable juices, etc.)

With these particular foods, you are looking out for the following signs of allergy; again, this is not an exhaustive list, and if you have any concerns whatsoever, don't hesitate to call your doctor.

- » Diarrhoea or vomiting
- » Cough
- » Eczema
- » Difficulty breathing
- » Wheezing and shortness of breath
- » Itchy throat and tongue

- » Itchy skin or rash
- » Swollen lips and throat
- » Facial swelling
- » Runny or blocked nose
- » Sore, red and itchy eyes
- » Hives

Please bear in mind that some foods, mainly some fruits and vegetables, can cause a little bit of irritation around the mouth (called a contact reaction/irritation) which isn't an allergy. If this happens, keep a food diary, and don't offer that particular food again for a couple of days to assess any future reaction.

REACTION TIMINGS

Immediate allergy symptoms typically manifest within two hours of exposure, while delayed symptoms can occur within a broader timeframe, ranging from two to 72 hours.

It's crucial to be vigilant for signs of allergic reactions. Immediate symptoms may include hives, facial swelling, vomiting and difficulty breathing. If your baby exhibits any of these symptoms, seek immediate medical attention.

Delayed symptoms might include persistent diarrhoea, eczema flare-ups or recurrent vomiting. While these may not appear urgent, they still require attention, and consulting with a healthcare professional is recommended.

SYMPTOM TYPE	Immediate allergic reactions that require URGENT medical attention	Delayed allergic reactions that require medical attention
Common symptoms	Hives, facial swelling, difficulty breathing, wheezing and shortness of breath, vomiting, swollen lips and throat, itchy throat and tongue	Diarrhoea, eczema and runny or blocked nose.
Timeframe of onset	Within two hours	Between two and 72 hours after exposure

Always consult a healthcare professional for personalized medical advice if you observe any concerning symptoms during the weaning process.

HOW TO INTRODUCE ALLERGENS

For babies with no family history of allergies, and for whom no concerns have arisen in their first six months of consuming formula or breastmilk, you may not choose to take any specific steps to introduce allergens other than introducing them before 12 months. But if you are concerned that your baby has allergies, or if you, your partner or other children have allergies, then it can be sensible to take a more cautious approach.

» Consult medical advice before starting weaning or before offering an allergen

» Only offer one allergen a day in small quantities, and increase gradually

» Only provide one allergen at a time in one meal, unless it has already been successfully introduced

» Avoid offering a new allergen if your child is unwell and it may be more difficult to interpret symptoms

Once you have introduced an allergen and it has been tolerated, continue to offer it to avoid the risk of an allergy developing.

HELPFUL ALLERGY SWAPS

There has been a big leap forward in the availability of alternative products for those with allergies, and most of these are also suitable for babies. Below I will give you some swaps that are safe to use when preparing meals for your baby.

DAIRY

Alternatives to cow's milk include plant-based milk alternatives such as:

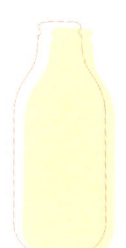

» Coconut milk
» Oat milk
» Soya milk

These can all be used in cooking, but should not be used as an alternative to breast or formula milk as a drink under the age of 12 months. It's best to avoid rice milk for young babies as these can contain arsenic. It is also best to avoid nut milks as these are low calorie. Choose options fortified with key vitamins like calcium and iodine where you can. You can also use breast milk in cooking, but it cannot be refrozen, so if you plan to do batch cooking, you cannot use previously frozen breast milk.

You can get great dairy-free yoghurts, and coconut yoghurt is another great swap.

EGGS

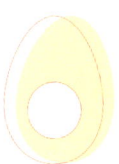

Health-food stores sell a specific product that you can use as a direct replacement for eggs. But if you can't get hold of this, there are some great swaps for eggs in cooking, and each will amount to the equivalent of 1 egg:

» 1 tablespoon flaxseed stirred into 3 tablespoons water (leave to stand for 5–10 minutes once combined)
» 1 tablespoon chia seeds and 80ml (3fl oz/⅓ cup) water
» ½ mashed banana (better for sweet recipes)
» 60ml (2fl oz/¼ cup) apple purée (sauce) (better for sweet recipes)
» 3 tablespoons peanut butter
» 60ml (2fl oz/¼ cup) soya yoghurt

NUTS

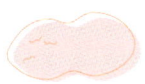

If your infant has been diagnosed with or is suspected of having a nut allergy, they will be referred to a medical professional specializing in allergies. During consultations with this professional, please take the opportunity to ask questions, ensuring you are clear on the safe management of your baby's allergy.

When it comes to nut alternatives, consider seed and granola butters. These alternatives mirror the creamy goodness of nut butter, offering a delightful swap without compromising taste or texture.

For a list of helpful allergy resources, see page 204.

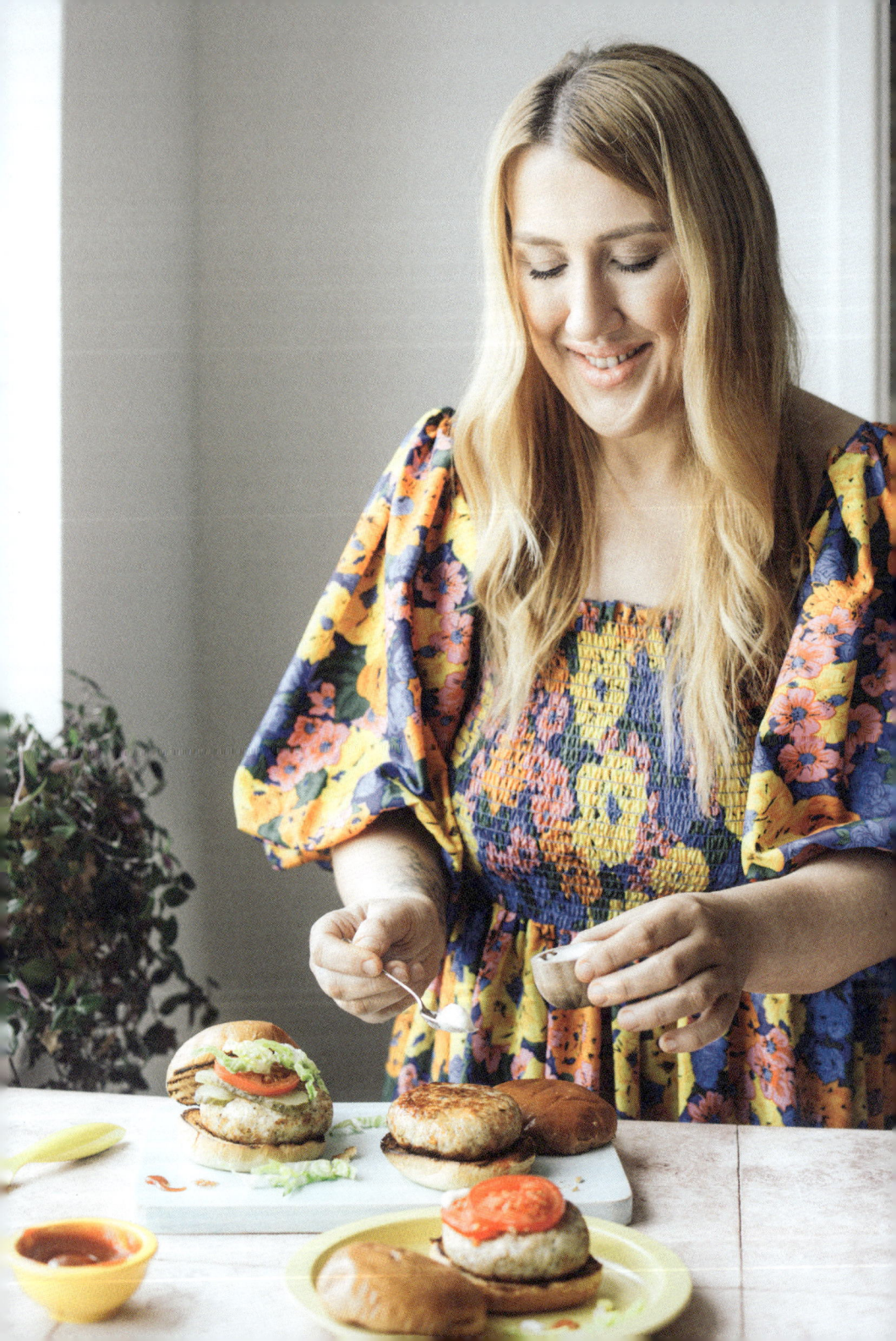

HOW TO PREPARE FOOD SAFELY

A baby's journey into the world of solid foods is an exciting and pivotal stage in their development. However, it does have its potential challenges, particularly regarding safety. A baby can choke on any food, but certain foods pose a more significant risk due to their size and shape.

Foods such as cherry tomatoes, olives, grapes and popcorn that are a similar shape and size to a baby's airway are particularly hazardous. These foods are going to be hard to dislodge and in extreme cases, they will require medical assistance to dislodge, which prolongs the period in which the baby is not breathing.

This is why it's vital to either cut foods so they are too large to be swallowed whole and require chewing, or so they are smaller than the airway and cannot get stuck.

When offering foods larger than the airway, ensure they are cooked until soft. Offering hard foods, such as raw apples, can be dangerous because a baby could bite off a hard chunk, which could then get lodged in the airway and cause the baby to choke. By ensuring the food is soft, you significantly reduce the choking risk. Because of this, we must teach our babies how to chew, and communicate why chewing is so important. We can help our baby learn to chew by eating as many meals as possible with them, and exaggerating our own chewing so they can watch and mimic our behaviour. You may feel silly doing this initially, but it's worth it.

I highly recommend my first aid course, run by Mini First Aid, which covers safe eating and CPR in depth. Check out the resources on page 204.

Overleaf is a guide for how to prepare and cook foods so they are safe for your baby. Please bear in mind that from approximately nine to ten months old, your baby will start practising their pincer grip, which is the art of picking up smaller foods between their forefinger and thumb. While practising this skill, they will most likely prefer foods cut into smaller pieces.

FRUIT	
Apple	1. Wash the apple well under cold water. 2. Cut in half and discard any seeds. 3. Slice each half into thick wedges. 4. Place into a microwave-safe bowl with a splash of water. 5. Microwave for 1–2 minutes until soft. 6. Serve once cooled.
Apricot	1. Select a very ripe apricot and wash it well under cold water. 2. Slice in half and discard the stone. 3. Cut each half into slices. 4. Serve.
Avocado	1. Select a ripe avocado. 2. Slice it in half and use a knife to carefully remove the stone. 3. Scoop the flesh away from the skin. 4. Cut the flesh into long, thick batons, about 2cm/¾in. 5. Serve.
Banana	1. Peel the banana. 2. Push down on the top of the banana so it naturally starts to split into three spears. 3. Serve the spears.
Blueberries	1. Wash the blueberries well under cold water. 2. Flatten the blueberries into discs with your thumb and forefinger, breaking the skin. 3. Serve.
Grapefruit	1. Use a sharp knife to slice the top and bottom off the grapefruit. 2. Using the same knife, peel off the skin, following the shape of the grapefruit. 3. Pull into segments, then remove the membrane and seeds. 4. Serve.
Grapes	1. Wash the grapes well under cold water. 2. Slice lengthways into quarters. 3. Serve.

Kiwi	1. Peel half of the kiwi so that your baby can hold the part with the skin on and suck/chew the peeled part. 2. Serve.
Mango	1. Wash the mango under cold water. 2. Cut the mango in half and remove the seed. 3. Cut each half into long, thick batons, about 2cm/¾in. 4. Serve.
Melon	1. Wash the melon well under cold water. 2. Use a sharp knife to remove the rind. 3. Slice the melon in half and remove the seeds. 4. Cut the flesh half into long, thick batons, about 2cm/¾in. 5. Serve.
Nectarine	1. Select a ripe nectarine and wash it well under cold water. 2. Slice it in half. 3. Carefully remove the stone. 4. Cut each half into long, thick batons, about 2cm/¾in. 5. Serve.
Orange	1. Peel the orange. 2. Pull into segments. 3. Remove the membrane and any pips. 4. Serve.
Passion fruit	1. Slice the passion fruit in half. 2. Scoop out the seeded pulp and mix into yoghurt. 3. Serve on a loaded spoon.
Peach	1. Select a ripe peach and wash it well under cold water. 2. Slice it in half. 3. Carefully remove the stone. 4. Cut each half into long, thick batons, about 2cm/¾in. 5. Serve.
Pineapple	1. Cut the top off the pineapple with a sharp knife. 2. Use the same sharp knife to remove the skin. 3. Slice the pineapple into 4 big chunks around and away from the core at the centre. 4. Cut the chunks into long, thick batons, about 2cm/¾in. 5. Serve.

Raspberries	1. Wash the raspberries well under cold water.
	2. Slice the raspberries in half lengthways and flatten slightly.
	3. Serve.
Ripe pear	1. Select a very ripe pear and wash it well under cold water.
	2. Top and tail the pear.
	3. Slice in half and discard any seeds.
	4. Cut each half into long, thick batons (use your index finger as a size guide).
	5. Serve.
Strawberries	1. Wash the strawberries well under cold water.
	2. Hull the strawberries by removing the green cap and stem.
	3. Serve.
Tangerine	1. Peel the tangerine.
	2. Divide into segments.
	3. Remove the membrane and any pips.
	4. Serve.
Watermelon	1. Wash the watermelon well under cold water.
	2. Slice the melon in half.
	3. Cut the flesh half into long, thick batons, about 2cm/¾in.
	4. Serve.

GRAINS	
Bread	1. Cut the bread into long, thick batons, about 2cm/¾in.
	2. Serve a few slices at a time.
Couscous	1. Cook the couscous according to the packet instructions.
	2. Stir in some yoghurt to thicken, so it's easier for baby to grab fistfuls. Alternatively, offer on a loaded spoon.
Noodles	1. Cook the noodles according to the packet instructions.
	2. Slice the noodles into 8cm (3in) strips.
	3. Serve a few pieces at a time.

| Pasta | 1. Cook the pasta according to the packet instructions – I recommend fusilli for easy gripping.
2. Serve whole, directly onto your baby's tray. |
| Rice | 1. Cook the rice for a little longer than the packet instructions recommend so it becomes sticky.
2. Serve directly onto your baby's tray or offer on a loaded spoon. |

MEAT	
Beef	1. Cook the beef as desired (see packaging for cooking options and instructions or speak to your butcher). It's okay for it to still be pink, as long as the internal temperature has reached at least 63°C/145°F. 2. Serve in long slices, about 2cm/¾in, removing any tough fat.
Chicken	1. Cook the chicken as desired (see packaging for cooking options and instructions or speak to your butcher), ensuring it is fully cooked through. 2. Serve in long slices, about 2cm/¾in.
Lamb	1. Cook the lamb as desired (see packaging for cooking options and instructions or speak to your butcher). It's okay for it to still be pink, as long as the internal temperature has reached at least 71°C/160°C. 2. Serve in long slices, about 2cm/¾in.
Pork	1. Cook the pork as desired (see packaging for cooking options and instructions or speak to your butcher), ensuring it is fully cooked through. 2. Serve in long slices, about 2cm/¾in.
Turkey	1. Cook the turkey as desired (see packaging for cooking options and instructions or speak to your butcher), ensuring it is fully cooked through. 2. Serve in long slices, about 2cm/¾in.

SEAFOOD	
Bass, cod, halibut and herring	1. Remove any bones from the fish. 2. Cook it all the way though (see packaging for cooking options or seek advice from your fishmonger). 3. Serve in long slices, about 2cm/¾in.
Salmon (fresh)	1. Remove any bones from the fish. 2. Cook it all the way though (see packaging for cooking options or seek advice from your fishmonger). 3. Serve in long slices, about 2cm/¾in.
Salmon (tinned)	1. Mash the tinned salmon into yoghurt or cream cheese. 2. Spread onto toast or rice cakes. 3. Serve in long slices, about 2cm/¾in.
Sardines (tinned)	1. Serve strips straight from the tin. 2. Alternatively, mash the tinned sardines into yoghurt or cream cheese and spread onto toast or rice cakes. 3. Serve in long slices, about 2cm/¾in.
Trout	1. Remove any bones from the fish. 2. Cook it all the way though (see packaging for cooking options or seek advice from your fishmonger). 3. Serve in long slices, about 2cm/¾in.
Tuna (fresh)	1. Remove any bones from the fish. 2. Cook it all the way through (see packaging for cooking options or seek advice from your fishmonger). 3. Serve in long slices, about 2cm/¾in.
Tuna (tinned)	1. Mash the tinned tuna into yoghurt or cream cheese. 2. Spread onto toast or rice cakes. 3. Serve in long slices, about 2cm/¾in.

VEGETABLES	
Asparagus	1. Wash the asparagus well under cold water. 2. Trim the dry ends. 3. Steam for 10 minutes. 4. Serve once cooled.
Aubergine (eggplant)	1. Wash the aubergine (eggplant) well under cold water. 2. Cut the top off and then cut the aubergine in half lengthways. 3. Cut each half into long, thick batons (use your index finger as a size guide). 4. Place onto a baking tray (sheet pan) and drizzle with vegetable oil. 5. Roast at 180°C/160°C fan/350°F/Gas mark 4 for 25–30 minutes. 6. Serve once cooled.
Broccoli	1. Wash the broccoli well under cold water. 2. Cut into florets. 3. Steam for 10 minutes. 4. Serve once cooled.
Butternut squash	1. Peel the butternut squash. 2. Cut in half lengthways and scoop out the seeds. 3. Cut each half into long, thick batons (use your index finger as a size guide). 4. Place onto a baking tray (sheet pan) and drizzle with vegetable oil. 5. Roast at 200°C/180°C fan/400°F/Gas mark 6 for 25–35 minutes. 6. Serve once cooled.
Carrot	1. Peel and cut into long, thick batons (use your index finger as a size guide). 2. Steam for 8–10 minutes. 3. Serve once cooled.
Cauliflower	1. Wash the cauliflower well under cold water. 2. Cut into florets. 3. Steam for 10 minutes. 4. Serve once cooled.

Celery	1. Wash the celery well under cold water.
	2. Cut the celery stick(s) in half.
	3. Place into a microwave-safe bowl with 2 tablespoons water.
	4. Microwave for 4–5 minutes.
	5. Serve once cooled.
Courgette (zucchini)	1. Wash the courgette (zucchini) well under cold water.
	2. Cut the top off and then cut the courgette in half lengthways.
	3. Cut each half into long, thick batons (use your index finger as a size guide).
	4. Place onto a baking tray (sheet pan) and drizzle with vegetable oil.
	5. Roast at 180°C/160°C fan/350°F/Gas mark 4 for 25–30 minutes.
	6. Serve once cooled.
Green beans	1. Wash the green beans well under cold water.
	2. Trim the ends.
	3. Steam for 8 minutes.
	4. Serve once cooled.
Mushrooms	1. Finely dice the mushrooms.
	2. Fry in 1 teaspoon of vegetable oil for 2–3 minutes.
	3. Stir into omelettes, fritters or mashed potato, or add to a cheese toastie
Parsnip	1. Peel the parsnip and remove the top.
	2. Cut into long, thick batons (use your index finger as a size guide).
	3. Place onto a baking tray (sheet pan) and drizzle with vegetable oil.
	4. Roast at 200°C/180°C fan/400°F/Gas mark 6 for 30–35 minutes.
	5. Serve once cooled.
Peas	1. Add the peas to a saucepan and cover with water.
	2. Bring the water to the boil and simmer for 3–4 minutes.
	3. Mash very slightly before serving to break the skin.
Pepper (bell pepper)	1. Wash the pepper well under cold water.
	2. Cut the pepper in half and deseed.
	3. Cut each half into long, thick batons (use your index finger as a size guide).
	4. Place onto a baking tray (sheet pan) and drizzle with vegetable oil.
	5. Roast at 180°C/160°C fan/350°F/Gas mark 4 for 25–30 minutes.
	6. Serve once cooled.

Potato	1. Wash the potato well under cold water. 2. Cut into long, thick batons (use your index finger as a size guide). 3. Place onto a baking tray (sheet pan) and drizzle with vegetable oil. 4. Roast at 200°C/180°C fan/400°F/Gas mark 6 for 30–35 minutes. 5. Serve once cooled.
Pumpkin	1. Cut the pumpkin into long, thick batons (use your index finger as a size guide). 2. Place onto a baking tray (sheet pan) and drizzle with vegetable oil. 3. Roast at 200°C/180°C fan/400°F/Gas mark 6 for 25–35 minutes. 4. Serve once cooled.
Sweetcorn (corn kernels)	1. Add the sweetcorn to a saucepan and cover with water. 2. Bring the water to the boil and simmer for 3–4 minutes. 3. Mash very slightly before serving to break the skin.
Sweet potato	1. Wash the sweet potato well under cold water. 2. Cut into long, thick batons (use your index finger as a size guide). 3. Place onto a baking tray (sheet pan) and drizzle with vegetable oil. 4. Roast at 200°C/180°C fan/400°F/Gas mark 6 for 30–40 minutes. 5. Serve once cooled.

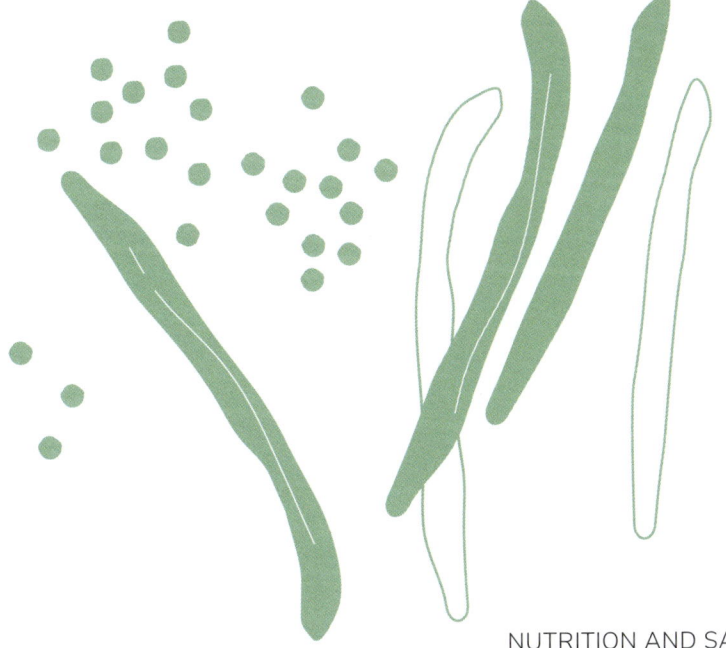

CHOKING VS GAGGING

A common concern regarding baby-led weaning is the issue of choking.

To set the record straight from the outset, it might surprise you that the likelihood of your baby choking on solid foods is no higher than with purées. The critical factor here is the texture and safe serving of the food, coupled with ensuring that your baby is developmentally prepared for the weaning process, as discussed on pages 20–21.

A likely and very common scenario during your baby's first few weeks of weaning is that they will gag. While this can be daunting to witness, it's entirely normal as your child learns how to eat and manipulate food in their mouth. Their gag reflex will diminish with time and experience with foods.

A baby who hasn't yet mastered swallowing food will use their gag reflex, located towards the front of their mouth, during the early stages. The gag reflex pushes food from the back of their mouth to the front as a natural inbuilt safeguard from choking.

A gagging baby often displays the following signs:
» Coughing
» Tongue thrusting forwards or out of their mouth
» Watery eyes
» A reddened face
» Vomiting

Although these symptoms can be disconcerting, they're entirely normal. A reassuring phrase like 'you can do it', 'work it out' or 'chew, chew' delivered in a composed and encouraging tone can help your baby resolve the situation. It's important to avoid attempting to scoop out the food with your fingers, as this can exacerbate the issue. While it's natural to feel alarmed, try to remain calm; a strong reaction could startle your baby, potentially causing them to swallow the food and choke.

Choking is very rare, but here are the signs to look out for:

» Sudden silence
» Rapid chest contraction as they try to draw in air
» A pale complexion
» Turning blue
» Loss of consciousness

You may notice that the signs of choking differ significantly from the previously mentioned gagging behaviours – almost the polar opposite in fact.

WHAT TO DO IF YOUR BABY CHOKES

If your baby starts choking, remove them from their highchair and administer decisive back blows between their shoulder blades. These back blows will often dislodge the obstructing food. If this does not work, ask someone nearby to call for an ambulance immediately. If the food does dislodge from the back blows, it's advisable to take your baby to A&E to be seen by a doctor as a precautionary measure.

I strongly recommend that all parents consider undergoing a first aid course before embarking on the weaning journey. I have a course available on my website (see page 204) designed to help parents feel fully equipped and confident to wean safely.

Getting Started

In the wonderful world of parenting, mealtimes are not just about sustenance; they're a journey of exploration, growth and discovery. Those precious moments spent around the family table are about more than simply fuelling your little one's body; they are building blocks for their future relationship with food.

As a parent, you hold the key to unlocking a world of flavours, textures and experiences that will shape your child's palate and relationship with food. Introducing your baby to solid foods is a pivotal moment in their development.

In this chapter, I won't just focus on the practical aspects of feeding. I'm here to support you on every step of a journey filled with messy moments, joyous discoveries and the promise of lifelong healthy eating habits. So buckle up – your adventure begins here!

ESSENTIAL TOOLS AND EQUIPMENT

You do not need to spend a lot of money on equipment for baby-led weaning, but there are certain essentials that every parent needs, such as a highchair.

That said, after weaning three children, I have discovered some nifty products that, while not essential, can make the experience more manageable. These products have stood the test of time (more than nine years) and still do their job well. I will share these product recommendations here, to help your BLW journey begin positively, minus too much mess!

HIGHCHAIR

When I started weaning Annabelle, I bought a beautiful wooden highchair that looked lovely in our little cottage, but the first time I used it, I knew we would not be friends. Annabelle sat in it awkwardly and proceeded to drop everything onto her lap, as the space between her and the tray was vast. For the rest of the week, I cursed the chair at least three times a day, and proceeded to trip over it every time I walked through the kitchen – it was HUGE!

By the time the weekend came, I'd already decided we would buy a more suitable highchair for our 'two up, two down' cottage – one that was a lot cheaper but did the job much better. To avoid making the same mistake, there are a few key things you should keep in mind when choosing a highchair.

EASE OF CLEANING

Picture the daily dance of mealtime messes and inevitable spills. Prioritize a highchair that simplifies your cleaning routine. Opt for a simple design, steering clear of intricate nooks and crannies. Fabric? A resounding no! Choose a highchair that doesn't just look clean but promises a hassle-free experience.

A FUTURE-READY DESIGN

Anticipate the evolving needs of your growing child. Will you want to remove the tray and bring your baby to the table in the future? Look for a highchair that seamlessly transitions from early feeding stages to more independent dining. Versatility should be a key feature, ensuring that the highchair remains a functional part of your child's journey beyond infancy.

A FOOTREST

Beyond mere comfort, a footrest provides stability, correct foot and leg positioning, improved concentration, reduced fatigue and enhanced hand-to-mouth coordination. A footrest isn't just a luxury; it's a fundamental component of a happy and successful weaning journey, supporting your baby's trunk and core. Having your child's feet on a footrest while sitting discourages slouching (sacral sitting), promotes stability and upright posture and helps minimize the risk of choking.

KITCHEN FRIENDLY DIMENSIONS

Consider the spatial dynamics of your kitchen. Choose a highchair that seamlessly integrates into your space without creating unnecessary clutter. The ideal highchair should complement your kitchen's aesthetics while providing a practical and comfortable solution for your baby's mealtimes.

FOLDABLE AND CONVENIENT STORAGE

Maximize your space by opting for a highchair that offers the convenience of folding and easy storage. This feature ensures that your highchair only monopolizes valuable space when in active use, making it a practical choice for compact and spacious kitchens.

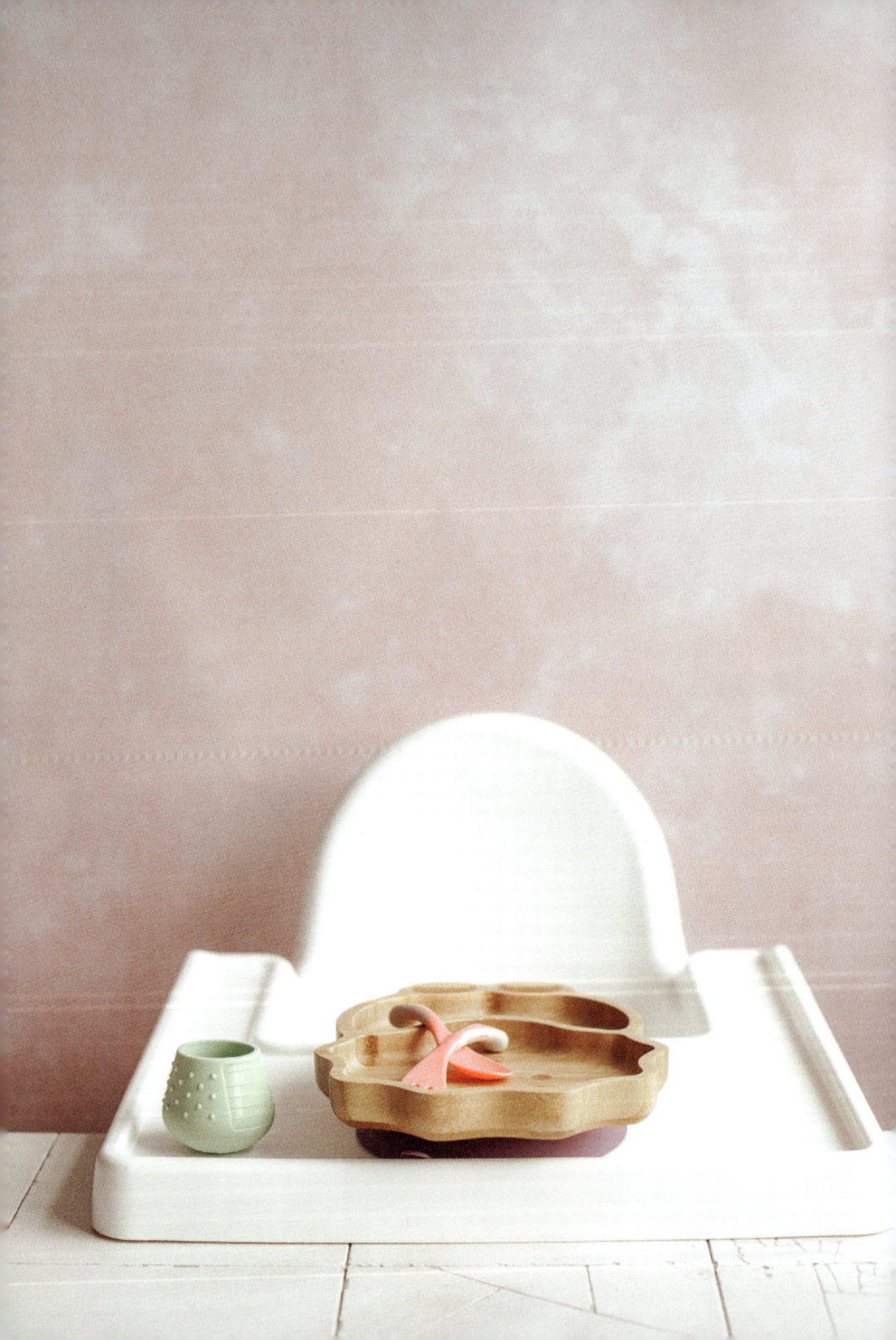

SUCTION MATS

When considering tableware, it's important to remember that unless you choose something that sticks to the highchair tray securely, the food you have lovingly prepared will likely end up on the floor within seconds. This is why I highly recommend opting for a suction mat. Suction mats comes in various sizes and colours, and offer a range of benefits:

» They stick very securely to plastic highchair trays and coated tables.

» They are easy to wash up and dishwasher-safe.

» You can find styles that fit most highchairs.

» Some version have lids, meaning leftovers can be taken on the go.

» Most are BPA-free (Bisphenol A, a chemical found in some plastics), but please check prior to purchasing.

CUTLERY

When venturing into the world of baby cutlery, choosing well-designed utensils is essential as proper cutlery plays a pivotal role in helping them master self-feeding. Opt for cutlery styles designed specifically for babies and young children. While many infant cutlery options mimic adult utensils with long handles, this can pose a challenge for small hands. Instead, I recommend selecting cutlery with short, ergonomic handles specifically shaped to facilitate a secure grip for little fingers. This ensures a comfortable and practical eating experience for your little one. What to consider when selecting cutlery:

» It has been tested and certified as safe.

» The handles are contoured to fit your infant's hand.

» It is made from food-safe materials.

» It is easy to clean and dishwasher-safe.

SPLASH MAT

A splash mat is a large PVC anti-slip mat that sits underneath your baby's highchair, protecting your floors and saving precious time when cleaning up. The mats are both waterproof and wipeable, and allow you to gather up all of your baby's dropped food and pour it directly into the bin.

There are some very pretty yet costly splash mats, but it's not worth spending a lot of money on unless you really want to. I do, however, recommend buying a mat designed specifically as a splash mat. Some people suggest using an old shower curtain or similar instead, but these are usually not made from anti-slip materials and may fail to prevent the highchair from toppling over.

Splash mats are also dual-use, and can also be used for:
» Messy play
» Garden play
» Potty training
» Indoor or outdoor picnics

A SMOCK BIB

A smock bib is a non-negotiable for BLW, offering practicality and peace of mind. Unlike traditional bibs, smock bibs provide extensive coverage, protecting your baby's entire front, shoulders and lap from inevitable spills and mess. Often crafted from easy-to-clean materials, these bibs minimize the post-meal clean-up effort for parents. Here are my tips for how to choose a good-quality smock bib:

» Look for a design that straps to the highchair to stop food from falling onto your baby's lap.
» Opt for a wipe-clean material.
» Ensure the material is wipeable between meals and also machine washable.
» Ensure the material is stain-resistant.

A good smock bib will not only protect clothes from being stained and prevent your water bill skyrocketing from numerous daily baths, but it may also save your sanity!

STARTING YOUR
WEANING JOURNEY

Some parents are happy to let their babies get fully stuck into meals with their hands or a loaded spoon, while others prefer a slower, steadier approach to weaning as they build their confidence. The recipes in this book cover all stages and approaches of the weaning journey.

Reflecting on my weaning journey with Annabelle back in 2015, the prevailing trend pushed by experts was to introduce one food at a time. Navigating the landscape of first-time motherhood and considering Annabelle's cow's milk allergy, I found comfort in this one-step-at-a-time approach.

Fast forward five years to weaning my twins, and a notable shift had occurred. My confidence was high and my approach more laid-back. Embracing the chaos of managing work, my daughter's homework and running a business, I found it more manageable to just serve my twins smaller portions of our family meals right from the start. It wasn't just a 90-degree turn; it was a complete 180!

You shouldn't feel pressured to follow a specific path; there is no right or wrong choice. In this chapter, I'll discuss various approaches so that you can determine which one is best for you and your baby at this time, or you might decide to make your own plan – it's entirely up to you.

Whatever you do, keep your expectations low. Your baby will view the food you offer like his or her toys, so don't be surprised if a lot of it ends up on the floor – this is very normal in the beginning.

METHOD 1: SLOW AND STEADY

For some parents, moving straight into meals is a step too far in the beginning. They may find the mess overwhelming or struggle to fit in the time for specific meals. So another approach in those early days is to stick to finger foods, offering strips of finger-width foods your baby can pick up and hold easily. This is great for developing fine motor skills and is excellent when eating out and eating on the go.

With this slow and steady approach, most parents offer finger food daily for the first month. After a month, you can slowly introduce meals at a pace that feels comfortable for you, working towards three meals a day by the age of 12 months. And if you prefer to follow this for less than a month, go ahead and do whatever works best for you.

It is entirely up to you how many servings of finger food you offer per week. I have suggested a simple plan below, which has been helpful to parents I have worked with, but again, please feel free to adapt.

» **Week 1: 1 offering a day**
» **Week 2: 2 offerings a day**
» **Week 3 and 4: 3 offerings a day**

Please remember that there is no right or wrong, and it's best to always follow your gut and do whatever feels right for you and your baby. At this stage, they will still be getting the nutrients they need from breast milk or formula (see page 22).

Below is a list of 50 finger food suggestions that are simple and easy to prepare for those taking this approach. You will find recipes for many of these in the recipe section.

FRUITS AND VEGETABLES

Sweet potato wedges
Roasted parsnip
Roasted carrot
Avocado slices rolled in breadcrumbs
    (for non-slip gripping)
Pineapple
Broccoli florets
Cauliflower florets
Steamed celery sticks
Roasted aubergine (eggplant)
    sticks

Roasted pepper strips
Green beans, steamed or toasted
Celeriac (celery root) wedges
Overripe pear wedges
Banana, quartered
Mango slices
Cucumber sticks
Mushrooms rolled in breadcrumbs
    (for non-slip gripping)
Roasted courgette (zucchini)
Roasted pumpkin wedges

BREAKFAST FOODS

Toast strips
Baked oats in strips
Oat cookies in strips
Fruit loaf in strips
Pancakes in strips
Waffle strips
Bagel slices
Crumpet slices
Banana/apple
French toast slices
English muffin slices

LUNCHES AND DINNERS

Toasted wrap slices
Omelette strips
Savoury muffin strips
Pinwheel strips
Quesadilla strips
Savoury fritter strips
Fish cake strips
Frittata slices
Mini quiche slices
Mini pizza slices
Strips of roasted chicken
Potato rösti slices

METHOD 2: DIVE STRAIGHT IN

The most popular BLW approach is to dive straight into feeding your baby family meals from day one – a relaxed, no-faff approach. With this method, you offer your baby a smaller portion of your own meals from six months onwards. You can start with one meal a day or jump straight into two or three meals per day.

If you're starting with one meal a day, lunch can be the easiest to begin with, as you can be flexible with timing it around naps. From this one meal, you will build up to three meals a day by 10–12 months. Many parents I work with decide to dive into three meals a day from six months, and if that feels right for you, then go for it.

The significant benefit to this approach is that it requires less preparation (and therefore much less brain power) because you are not having to organize a separate meal for your baby – which is always handy when you're running on little sleep, as many parents often are.

METHOD 3: FLEXIBLE

Although I have outlined two approaches you could take, feel free to devise your own plan. You could perhaps start with breakfast in month one, lunch in month two and dinner in month three. It's also okay to just go with the flow and decide as you go along.

You may start slow and then discover that your confidence is higher than you anticipated, and so decide to dive straight into meals. Or the opposite may happen: you may plunge directly into meals and then pull back and take a slower approach because things are feeling a tad overwhelming.

The most important thing is to create a calm, relaxed environment where you and your baby feel happy and confident.

THE IMPORTANCE OF WATER

Introducing a sippy cup or a small open cup of water from the start is key, regardless of your chosen weaning approach.
Be prepared to experiment with various cup styles to find what suits your baby best. Initially, offering small sips from an open cup might be beneficial until your little one gets the hang of the sippy cup independently.

Tap water is perfectly suitable. However, avoid bottled water due to the potential high mineral and salt content.

While there's no strict water consumption quota, helping your baby to drink until they are comfortable and proficient with their sippy cup ensures hydration needs are met.

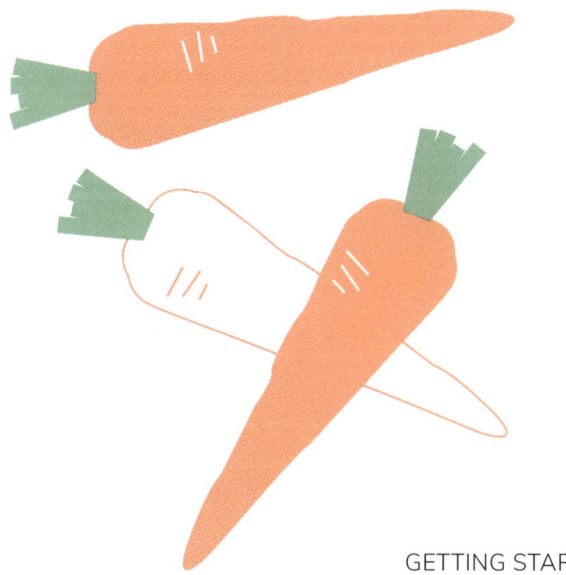

MANAGING THE MESS

I've heard people joke about the mess that comes at the start of baby-led weaning. I must admit, as someone who was weaning twins during the pandemic while home-schooling their daughter, the mess of weaning and the general lack of time to clean and tidy my house did have a massive impact on my mental health. Everyone reacts differently to mess, but I'm not too fond of it. 'A tidy home equals a tidy mind' is the motto I live by. Below I have outlined some strategies I found helpful to manage messy mealtimes.

THE OUTSIDE BIN

I've found that throwing food directly into the kitchen bin, without spilling half of it around the bin, is a little tricky! So I keep my large outside rubbish bin by my back kitchen door so I can shake off bibs and splash mats without the fear of giving myself more to clean up.

A SPLASH MAT

Instead of crawling around on your hands and knees, picking up your baby's mess, you can grab the mat by its corners and take it straight to the outdoor bin. Once shaken off, give it a quick wipe, and it's ready for your baby's next meal.

A SMOCK BIB

As discussed on page 66, a smock bib is a godsend when managing messy mealtimes. If you carefully remove the bib before taking your baby out of their highchair, you can take it to the bin to shake it off, preventing all of the food remnants from falling onto the floor as you lift your baby out.

A HIGHCHAIR HOOK

A nifty way to keep your kitchen a little less cluttered is to attach a stick-on hook to the back of your baby's highchair to hold your baby's smock bib and a bag of wipes.

GO ALFRESCO

If, like me, you live in the UK and expect rain most days, then you may roll your eyes at this one. However, I encourage you to eat outside at every opportunity. As well as being a fun change of scene, you don't risk getting spaghetti Bolognese plastered on your walls when you're in the garden!

KEEP PORTIONS SMALL

This may seem obvious, but I have been that parent who has piled their children's plates sky high like they were my own, forgetting their tummies are much smaller than mine. Keeping portions small is an easy way to limit the mess, and also avoid your baby becoming overwhelmed by the amount of food in front of them. By offering small portions, there is less for your baby to throw! You can of course top up your baby's plate as needed, but starting with a big pile of noodles could be a recipe for disaster.

And to the parents in the thick of it who are not coping with the mess – it's okay to admit that you're not enjoying it. When I had down days, I would try my best to focus on the end goal and remind myself of the benefits and why I chose BLW in the first place. Please remember that your baby will not be messy forever; a time will come when they are eating with a fork and spoon, and you will feel very proud of your baby and yourself for not giving up.

COMBATING COMMON HURDLES

In this section we will explore some of the common hurdles parents experience during the weaning process, from lack of interest in food, to food throwing and fussy eating. These challenges aren't just my own; they echo the shared experiences of the incredible parents I've had the privilege to work with.

Reflecting on my own journey, there's a sense that knowing then what I know now might have softened the bumps in the road – those tricky phases of food throwing and fussy eating with my eldest. Yet, as daunting as they were, those very challenges led me to seek expert advice, gifting me the profound understanding I carry today.

I hope the information given here transforms challenges into shared, manageable moments, shaping a weaning experience that's not just about hurdles but about the beautiful, messy dance of discovery between parents and their little ones.

LACK OF INTEREST

I often get messages from worried parents with babies ranging from around six to eight months old who have no interest in food. They feel flat, anxious and full of worry. When these messages appear, I firstly reassure the parent that this is normal behaviour and that they are not doing anything wrong. There can be a temptation to switch to purées in this situation, but that isn't always the answer.

Firstly, step back and remember that all babies are very different. Having twins, I see this every day. When you just have one baby, you can't see that while your baby works on one milestone, another baby born on the same day focuses on a different one. They will both achieve all of their milestones eventually, but in differing orders. Our job as parents is to give our babies the tools and opportunities they need to work on these milestones, but unfortunately, we can't do the work for them, nor can we control the order in which they work on them or the date they achieve them.

To strengthen and support your baby's interest in food, I have created a list of tips to help you encourage your baby on their journey:

1. **Timing:** Offer food at the right time, when your baby isn't too hungry or too full of milk. About 1½ hours after a milk feed is ideal.
2. **Keep them company:** Sit with your baby and, as much as possible, eat what they are eating so they can watch how you do it and see that it's safe.
3. **Small portions:** Offer just a couple of pieces of food at a time so they don't become too overwhelmed.
4. **Tiredness:** Make sure you aren't offering solids when they are too tired. It's hard work to eat solid food early on, and they will give up quickly if they don't have the energy.
5. **Switch sittings:** If the meal you are offering isn't working, try another; so if you're offering breakfast and they aren't taking to it, try lunch, or vice versa.

Weaning shouldn't be scary or stressful; we put a lot of pressure on ourselves and our babies, but they will all get there eventually, I promise!

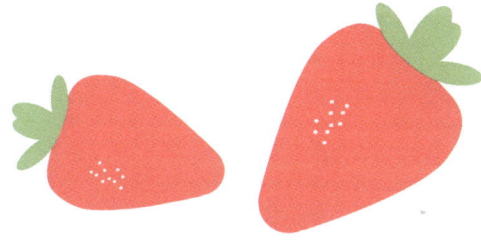

FOOD THROWING

Nothing is more exasperating than when your baby suddenly transforms into an Olympic javelin thrower during mealtimes. The urge to retrieve the discarded food from the floor and launch it right back at them might seem appealing (come on, am I the only one?), but it's safe to say that this approach might not yield the best results in dealing with such behaviour.

Let's explore some more sensible tactics to combat frustrating food throwing:

1. **Small portions:** Avoid overloading your baby's plate. This both keeps them from feeling overwhelmed and reduces the ammunition they have for their throwing endeavours.
2. **Strategic side plate:** Keep a separate side plate handy. When you sense your baby is on the brink of launching a food missile, calmly suggest they place the food on the side plate instead.
3. **Uninterrupted focus:** Disregard the hurling antics and continue your meal as if nothing has happened. Sometimes, a lack of attention can curb the appeal.
4. **Silent clean-up:** If your baby is in the same room during the mealtime clean-up, discreetly pick food up without uttering a word. This approach sends a message without adding fuel to the fire.
5. **Elevated exit:** If the throwing spree persists, gently remove the bib or any mealtime paraphernalia, lower your child to the floor, and calmly state, 'Looks like you're all done for today.' Set aside the uneaten food in case they have a sudden change of heart and realize they really do want to sit and eat, rather than sit and throw! They'll recognize the need to cease throwing if their hunger kicks in.
6. **Distraction tactics:** If none of the above work, try distracting your baby away from throwing food with a new plate or new mealtime environment – perhaps remove the highchair tray and put your baby up to the table, or have a picnic in the living room or garden if it's a nice day.

As hard as it is, the best thing you can do is remain calm, ignore when you can and not draw too much attention to the behaviour. As babies get older, they start to recognize that their actions can result in reactions from their parents and caregivers, and they can play on that fact. Babies and toddlers have very little autonomy and control, and how much they eat is sometimes the only thing that is their choice. Throwing is just another example of them exercising that choice – try not to let it become a battle.

HIGHCHAIR HURDLES

As your toddler grows, you might notice a significant shift in their dining preferences, and one common challenge parents face is the reluctance to sit in a highchair. Engaging in a power struggle over this issue is unlikely to result in a peaceful mealtime, let alone a well-fed child. Instead, consider some alternative strategies to keep both your child and your sanity intact.

If your toddler resists the highchair, don't push the issue. Forcing them into it is likely to be counterproductive and may not lead to any meaningful resolution. Instead, adapt to their changing preferences and create a more relaxed dining environment. Try having an indoor picnic in the living room, though do be prepared with a splash mat on the floor and plenty of towels and baby wipes on hand to manage any spills.

When my daughter reached her first birthday, the highchair began to gather dust as she transitioned into a grazer. She preferred nibbling throughout the day, often on the move. Whether it was munching on sandwiches on the sofa or enjoying apples while strolling through the park, her newfound eating style became our new normal. This change allowed us to adopt a more flexible schedule, which was actually a welcome relief.

FUSSY EATING

The variety of foods we offer and how we communicate to our babies during the first six months of weaning can impact their long-term behaviours and support the prevention of fussy eating habits from forming.

If you are worried about your baby turning into a fussy eater or experiencing fussy eating phases in the future, don't panic. So many things can help prevent this behaviour – or manage it when already present – and I will cover them in this section.

As a bit of background and reassurance, Annabelle hit the fussy eating stage at around 14 months, but gradually she returned to eating everything she loved as a baby. The only food she doesn't like to this day is hard-boiled egg, and this is ironic because, looking back, I didn't offer her eggs as a baby because I had a severe dislike of them myself. Now, I wish I'd read this book and listened to my own advice!

EASE THE PRESSURE

Another important tip is to keep mealtimes calm and relaxed; you don't want to associate any emotional attachment, pressure or reward towards food. This means taking a very laid-back approach to what your baby does and does not eat, keeping conversations away from food, not encouraging them to eat more and avoiding any emotional reaction to food eaten or not eaten.

The approach should be: 'This is your meal. It's up to you if you eat it.' If they eat it, we don't praise them; if they don't, we don't express anger or disappointment.

This approach is vital because fussy eating is more often than not linked to developmental changes – for example a desire for autonomy or control – rather than food. As our children have very little control over their lives, they crave it, so when they notice that they can cause an emotional reaction, whether good or bad, by not eating, they will enjoy the power. It's only by taking the reaction away and allowing your child to realize that their behaviour will not elicit a specific outcome, that things can start to change.

VARIETY

As discussed on page 32, the best tip I can give any parent starting to wean is to offer your baby as much variety as possible before their first birthday, including foods you don't like yourself. My experience with Annabelle is a prime example of why this is so important. Doing this will make your soon-to-be toddler feel safe and comfortable with a variety of different foods and reduce the likelihood of picky eating.

PORTION SIZES

Finally, I suggest keeping portions sizes very small. It's easy to forget how tiny our babies' tummies are, and offering a big plate of food can overwhelm them. The great thing about offering less is that you can always add more!

I understand this is a lot of information to digest, so here is an overview of how I suggest approaching mealtimes to prevent fussy eating habits from forming:

» Keep mealtimes calm and relaxed.
» Offer no praise for food eaten.
» Show no anger or disappointment for food not eaten.
» Do not bribe or encourage your baby to eat more.
» Place no expectations on your baby to eat.
» Keep conversations away from the topic of food.
» Keep portion sizes small to avoid overwhelming your baby.

Finally, please remember that just because your child doesn't eat something when it is first offered, it doesn't mean they never will. Familiarity brings a lot of comfort, and exposure is critical here. Eat together – and eat the same things – as much as you can. This removes some of the fear of the unknown for babies and creates good habits.

If you find that your baby or toddler is consistently consuming a limited variety of foods, leading to heightened stress during mealtimes, it's advisable to seek assistance from a professional. They can provide guidance and support to help you navigate and overcome these challenges.

EATING OUT

One of the things I loved about baby-led weaning was eating a warm meal while eating out, as I didn't have to sit and spoon-feed my baby! Most restaurants are very baby-friendly and won't mind you bringing food in for your baby, or if you want or need (both very valid) a break, then you can usually find something on the restaurant menu you can share with your little one.

Here are a few things you might like to consider taking with you when eating out to ensure you can enjoy a stress-free meal:

A BOOSTER SEAT

Most restaurants will have highchairs, but grabbing one on a busy weekend or during the school holidays can be tricky. There's also the annoyance of not all highchairs having trays or being far too big for your little one at the start of your weaning journey.

You may like to take a booster seat with you for peace of mind. These attach safely to a regular chair and have a tray included.

A SUCTION PLATE

If you prefer putting your little one's food on a tray, suction plates are very light and compact to transport. You can find plates that have lids, too, so you can always pack food at home and take it with you. And if you're sharing food, any leftovers can be safely stored for later.

A SMOCK BIB

The smock bib is an excellent coverall to keep your baby clean when eating out. It's also light and compact for your changing bag.

A BAG FOR MESSY BITS

When you're out of the house, you obviously won't have easy access to your laundry basket, so take a handy plastic bag to put all the messy bits in.

TOYS

I recommend bringing toys to keep little ones occupied when eating out, whether it's baby books, a quiet activity toy or, when older, magic painting books or a small sticker book. Anything to help fill that gap between ordering and getting your food, which can feel endless!

ORDERING FOR BABY

When eating out with your baby, some parents find it convenient to bring items from home, with a bento-style box being an excellent choice due to its multiple watertight compartments that can accommodate liquids and yoghurts.

Alternatively, if you desire a break from meal preparation, consider selecting a meal suitable for both you and your baby, fostering a shared dining experience. In such cases, avoiding excessive salt intake for the rest of the day is advisable to ensure your baby stays within the recommended daily limit of 1g.

Another engaging option is a pick-and-mix approach, allowing your baby to sample a variety of tastes and textures by sharing small portions from your and your fellow diners' plates.

DO WHAT YOU NEED TO DO

I mentioned bringing toys to keep your kids occupied while you wait for food. However, I want to be honest in this book, parent to parent. Sometimes, this just won't cut the mustard. Sometimes, you have to wait longer than expected and the toys get boring.

As I write this, my twin boys are still very much in the tantrum phase, and although some parents will not agree with this approach, when needed, I will let my boys watch a cartoon on my phone when eating out. The way I see it, I'd rather have a few judgmental stares than my toddlers kicking off and our food becoming cold.

Toys are great, but when necessary, feel free to bring the screen out if it helps.

Recipe
Know-how

In the whirlwind of modern family life, where every moment counts, nourishing your baby with wholesome, homemade meals can feel daunting. That's precisely why this cookbook focuses on simplicity and efficiency. Each recipe is designed to be ready in 20 minutes or less, ensuring your baby-led weaning (BLW) journey is as stress-free as possible.

Whether you're an experienced home cook in search of quick and nutritious family meals, or a kitchen novice eager to learn, this collection of 60 easy recipes caters for all ages, with a particular emphasis on your little one's developing palate.

Before we dive into the recipes, I have included some helpful advice on stocking your kitchen with food essentials and basic equipment, freezing and reheating foods, and my favourite handy hacks.

Prepare to delight in watching your baby discover the joys of food without it eating into your precious time.

ESSENTIAL INGREDIENTS

Picture this: you're in the middle of crafting a delicious homemade meal for your baby, when suddenly you find yourself stuck without a key ingredient. We've all been there, and it can be frustrating. That's why I've put together this handy list of pantry, fresh and frozen essentials.

This is an excellent opportunity to sort through your cupboards and make a note of what you already have and what you will need. You can then supplement your essentials with seasonal fruit and vegetables and fresh produce.

PANTRY ESSENTIALS

Baking goods
Baking powder
Unsweetened cocoa
    powder
Desiccated (dried
    shredded) coconut
Dried breadcrumbs
Ground almonds
Plain (all-purpose) flour
Self-raising
    (self-rising) flour
Vanilla essence

Cereals
Oats

Dairy
Unsalted butter or
    dairy-free alternative

Herbs
Dried basil
Dried oregano
Dried parsley
Mixed herbs

Oils
Olive oil
Vegetable oil

Pasta, Rice and Noodles
Basmati rice
Dried egg noodles
Fusilli pasta
Microwave rice pouches
Orzo

Sauces and Pastes
Passata
Red curry paste
Thai curry paste
Green pesto
Red pesto
Reduced-salt
    soya sauce

Snacks
Unsalted rice cakes

Spices
Ground allspice
Ground cinnamon
Ground cumin
Mild chilli powder
Mild curry powder
Smoked paprika

Spreads and Syrups
Lemon curd
Low-sugar jam
Maple syrup
Smooth peanut butter

Stocks
Low-salt beef stock
    (bouillon) cubes

Low-salt chicken stock
    (bouillon) cubes
Low-salt vegetable stock
    (bouillon) cubes

Tins
Chickpeas (garbanzos)
    in water
Chopped tomatoes

Coconut cream or milk
Green lentils in water
Low salt and sugar
    baked beans
Red kidney beans
    in water
Tomato purée (paste)
Tinned tuna

FRESH PRODUCE

Bakery
Tortilla wraps
White bread

Dairy and Eggs
Full-fat Greek yoghurt
    or dairy-free
    alternative
Full-fat cream cheese
    or dairy-free
    alternative

Full-fat milk or dairy-
    free alternative
Medium eggs
Cheddar cheese or
    dairy-free alternative

Fruit
Apples
Bananas
Mixed berries
Pears

Vegetables
Baking potatoes
Cherry tomatoes
Onions
Red (bell) peppers
Carrots
Garlic
Ginger
Broccoli
Cauliflower
Sweet potato

FROZEN PRODUCE

Meat
Chicken breasts
Minced (ground)
    beef
Minced (ground)
    chicken
Minced (ground)
    lamb

Pastry
Ready-rolled puff
    pastry

Fruit
Frozen blueberries
Frozen mango
Frozen mixed berries
Frozen strawberries

Vegetables
Frozen broccoli
Frozen butternut
    squash chunks
Frozen cauliflower
Frozen mixed vegetables
Frozen peas
Frozen spinach
Frozen sweetcorn

RECOMMENDED KITCHEN EQUIPMENT

Whether you're an experienced home cook or just starting to explore the world of cooking for your little one, my recommended equipment checklist will help you make informed choices about what will be most useful to have on hand to ensure food prep is stress-free.

» 12-hole mini-muffin tray
» 20cm (8in) cake tins x 2
» 900g (2lb) loaf tin
» Baking tray (sheet pan) x 2
» Chopping (cutting) board x 2
» Colander
» Food processor or blender
» Frying pan (skillet)
» Grater
» Measuring jug (pitcher)
» Mixing bowl x 2
» Ovenproof dish x 2
» Roasting tray
» Saucepan x 3
» Sharp knife x 2
» Spatula
» Weighing scales or measuring cups – I find cups so much quicker and easier to use, but you'll find both measurements included in this book
» Wooden spoon x 2

HANDY KITCHEN HACKS

As a devoted home cook myself, I know the joy of preparing meals for my family, but I also understand that life is a balancing act. Cooking should be enjoyable, not overwhelming, as it can be when you're juggling a multitude of responsibilities. From time-saving strategies to ingredient substitutions and clever shortcuts, these hacks are tailored to simplify your time in the kitchen, ensuring a manageable and calm environment while also elevating your confidence and expertise in preparing meals your baby will adore.

WEEKLY MEAL PLANNING

Investing in a meal planner, whether this be a trusty notebook or a convenient magnetic fridge chart, can be a game-changer in your culinary endeavours. Not only does it help with planning the week ahead, it also prevents you from purchasing unnecessary items during your food shop and therefore saves you money (you might be surprised how much!).

With a meal planner, you can stay on top of your food cupboard or pantry inventory, making the most of your freezer stash. But the most rewarding aspect is the sense of calm and organization it brings to your life. There will be no more frantic, last-minute meal decisions; you'll be well prepared to tackle the days ahead.

EVENING PREPPING

If, like mine, your children crave your attention and prefer cuddles to cot naps, then a little evening prep is a strategy that can significantly reduce your stress levels. Take a look at the suggestions overleaf.

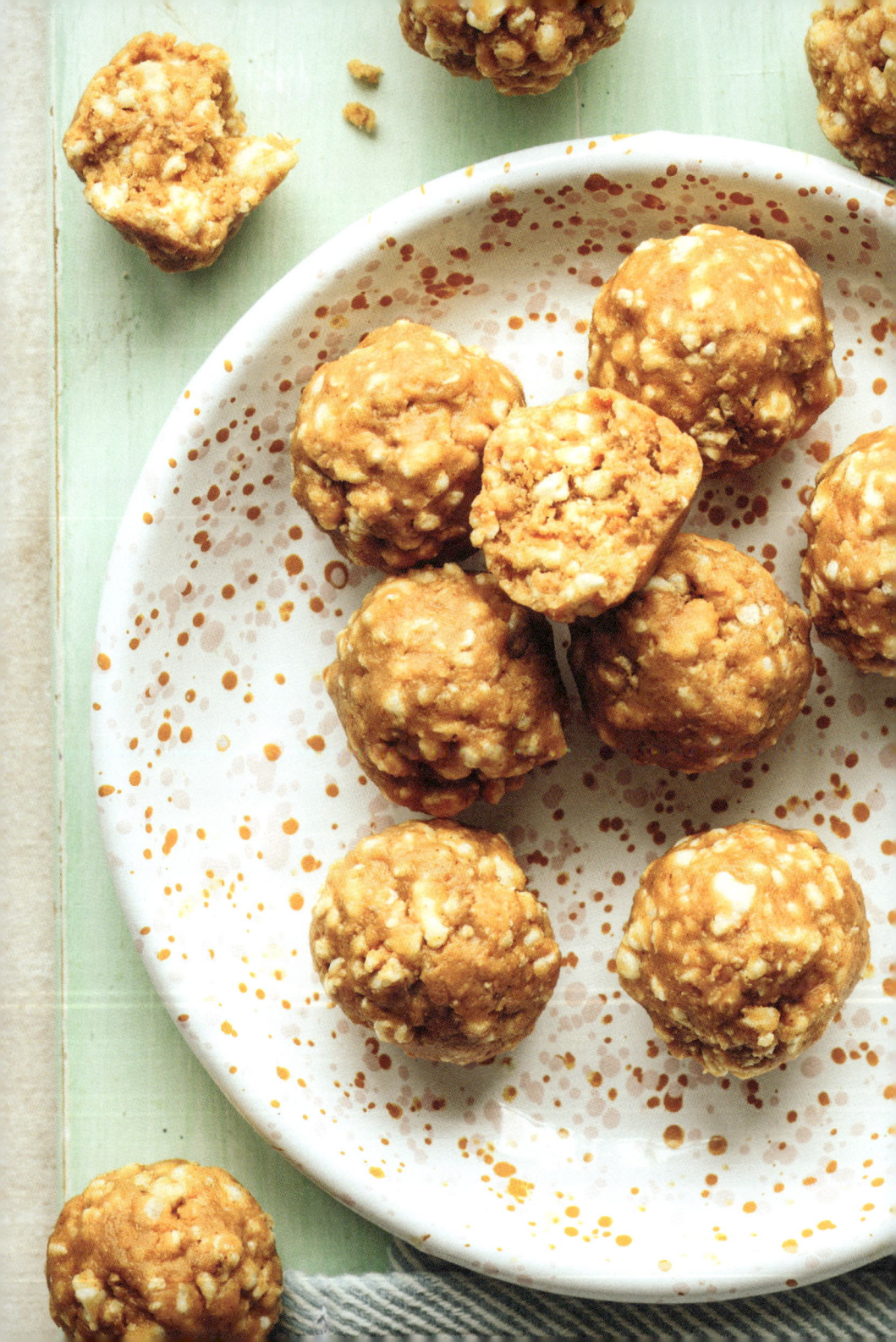

Breakfast

» Lay out bowls and spoons on the breakfast table.
» Place cereal boxes on the breakfast table if this is your desired breakfast choice.
» Take pancakes or breakfast muffins from the freezer and place them in the fridge to defrost overnight.

Lunch

» Prepare packed lunches, regardless of whether you'll eat out or stay in.
  OR
» Retrieve leftovers/meals from the freezer and transfer them to the fridge to defrost.

Dinner

» Slice all the meats and vegetables for tomorrow's main meal, storing them in airtight containers in the fridge.
  OR
» Take a slow-cook 'dump bag' or frozen meal out of the freezer and let it thaw in the fridge overnight.

DUMP BAGS

Dump bags are a convenient meal preparation method whereby ingredients for a slow-cooker recipe are pre-assembled, stored in a bag and then 'dumped' into the slow cooker for an easy and time-saving meal. The beauty of this method is that it allows you to reclaim precious time while your baby is awake and clamouring for your attention. And even if you do find pockets of time to prep while your little one plays nearby or naps, other tasks will likely demand your attention, such as work, cleaning, tidying or taking a well-deserved break.

BATCH COOKING

When it comes to savvy time management in the kitchen, batch cooking reigns supreme. Since you're already in the process of making a meal, why not double or triple the ingredients and create extra portions for your freezer stash and future meals? The brilliance of batch cooking lies in its simplicity – you don't need to adjust cooking times; you simply increase the quantity of the ingredients.

This approach minimizes your time spent cooking and ensures that you have a treasure trove of ready-made meals at your fingertips. It's a win-win scenario that simplifies your BLW journey while allowing you to savour every moment with your little one.

THE MAGIC OF ICE-CUBE TRAYS

Ice-cube trays are your unsung heroes when it comes to meal preparation. They offer a convenient way to portion and store various ingredients, and their small, uniform compartments make them perfect for freezing sauces. Here's how to make the most of them.

SAUCES
Homemade sauces such as pasta sauces are a breeze to make, but we often prepare more than we need. Instead of letting those delicious leftovers go to waste, follow these simple steps to freeze them efficiently:

» **Prepare your sauce:** Start by making your favourite pasta sauce. Whether it's a classic tomato sauce or a vibrant pesto, prepare and cook it according to your recipe.
» **Cool to room temperature:** If the sauce is hot, let it cool to room temperature. This step is crucial to prevent condensation inside the ice-cube trays.
» **Portion into ice-cube trays:** Carefully pour the sauce or pesto into the compartments of your clean ice-cube trays.

Leave a small gap at the top to allow for expansion as the sauce freezes.
» **Cover and freeze:** Place the ice-cube trays in the freezer, ensuring they are level to prevent spills. Cover the trays with cling film (plastic wrap) to protect the sauce from other items in the freezer.
» **Pop and store:** Once the sauce cubes are frozen solid, usually within a few hours, remove them from the ice-cube trays and transfer them to a resealable freezer bag. Remember to name and date the bag to keep track of freshness.

Do not freeze for any longer than 3 months.

USING YOUR FROZEN SAUCES
Now that you've mastered the art of freezing sauces and pesto in ice-cube trays, it's time to put these little flavour bombs to use. Here are some quick and easy meal ideas:
» **Pasta perfection:** Stir a couple of frozen pasta or pesto sauce cubes into freshly cooked pasta and warm over a low heat until the sauce has melted and coated the pasta thoroughly.
» **Veggie boost:** Add a pesto cube to steamed or roasted vegetables for an instant burst of flavour and nutrients.
» **Pizza night:** Use tomato sauce cubes as a base for homemade pizzas.
» **Dips and spreads:** Thaw a sauce cube to use as a dip or spread to accompany baby-friendly finger foods.
» **Soup enhancer:** Stir tomato sauce cubes into tomato-based soups to enhance them, or add a basil pesto cube to a creamy soup for a fresh twist.

By incorporating this ingenious freezing method into your BLW routine, you'll save time and reduce food waste while ensuring that your baby enjoys a variety of delicious and nutritious meals. Say goodbye to kitchen stress and hello to culinary convenience with frozen pasta sauce cubes always at your disposal.

THE BRILLIANCE OF FROZEN FRUITS AND VEGETABLES

As we continue our journey through the world of BLW, it's time to uncover another ingenious hack that will revolutionize your meal preparation: the use of frozen fruits and vegetables. While fresh produce is undeniably excellent, frozen options come with many benefits that can simplify your BLW adventure and enhance the nutritional value of your little one's meals.

YEAR-ROUND AVAILABILITY

One of the most significant advantages of using frozen fruits and vegetables is their year-round availability. Regardless of the season, you can always access a wide variety of frozen produce options in your local supermarket. This means you can incorporate diverse flavours and nutrients into your baby's diet, even when certain fruits and vegetables are out of season or not readily available.

CONVENIENCE

Pre-prepared frozen fruits and vegetables are incredibly convenient for busy parents. They're often already washed, peeled, chopped and ready to use, saving precious time in the kitchen. No more peeling and dicing carrots; grab what you need from your freezer and you're good to go.

NUTRIENT RETENTION

Contrary to popular opinion, frozen fruits and vegetables are often just as nutritious, if not more so, than their fresh counterparts. This is because they are typically frozen at the peak of ripeness, when their nutrient content is at its highest. The freezing process locks in these nutrients, ensuring your baby gets the maximum nutritional benefit from every bite.

REDUCED FOOD WASTE

Frozen produce is handy when you need only a single portion of a fruit or vegetable. There's no need to worry about the rest going to waste. This is especially helpful when preparing small meals for your baby, as you can avoid the guilt of discarding unused fresh produce.

COST-EFFECTIVE

Frozen fruits and vegetables are often more budget-friendly than their fresh counterparts, especially for out-of-season or exotic varieties. This means you can provide your baby with a diverse range of fruits and vegetables without breaking the bank.

LONGER SHELF LIFE

Unlike fresh produce, which has a limited shelf life, frozen fruits and vegetables can be stored for an extended period. They are less prone to spoilage and can be an essential part of your long-term meal-planning strategy.

QUICK AND EASY PREP

Frozen fruits and vegetables can be a lifesaver when you're short on time. They require minimal preparation – all you need to do is defrost or cook them according to your recipe. Whether adding them to oats or incorporating them into a main meal, the convenience factor cannot be underestimated.

These frozen gems are a valuable addition to your kitchen arsenal, offering convenience, nutrition and variety, and helping to make mealtimes a breeze for you and your little one. Say goodbye to seasonal limitations and hello to the year-round goodness of frozen produce.

STORAGE, FREEZING AND REHEATING GUIDELINES

Life as a parent can be unpredictable, and planning and preparing ahead is essential to maintain your sanity. Unless stated otherwise, all the recipes in this book can be safely stored in the refrigerator for up to 3 days, and, where freezable, can be frozen for up to 3 months. Below I explain how to safely freeze and reheat the recipes.

Important note: Don't refreeze something that has already been frozen, so only defrost what you plan to cook straightaway.

FRITTERS AND PANCAKES

Freezing:
Let the food cool thoroughly, then place on a baking tray (sheet pan) flat in the freezer for up to an hour. You can then transfer them into an airtight container or freezer bag. This will stop them sticking together. They will keep in the freezer for up to 3 months.

Defrosting:
Remove as many from the freezer as you need and defrost fully at room temperature for 2–3 hours, or overnight in the fridge.

Reheating:
Place the food in a frying pan on a low heat. Fry until piping hot throughout, about 2–3 minutes on each side.

PINWHEELS AND PASTRIES

Freezing:
I find pastry-based recipes are best frozen raw. Construct the pinwheels or pastries but don't bake them. Place the raw pastry on a baking tray (sheet pan) flat in the freezer for up to an hour. You can then transfer them into an airtight container or freezer bag. This will stop them sticking together. They will keep in the freezer for up to 3 months.

Defrosting:
Remove as many from the freezer as you need and defrost fully at room temperature for 2–3 hours, or overnight in the fridge.

Reheating:
Follow the cooking instructions in the recipe.

CAKES AND MUFFINS

Freezing:
Let the food cool thoroughly, then place on a baking tray (sheet pan) flat in the freezer for up to an hour. You can then transfer them into an airtight container or freezer bag. This will stop them sticking together. They will keep in the freezer for up to 3 months.

Defrosting:
Remove as many from the freezer as you need and defrost fully at room temperature for 2–3 hours, or overnight in the fridge.

Reheating:
Sprinkle with water and microwave on high for 20–30 seconds, or wrap in tin foil and bake in the oven at 180°C/160°C fan/350°F/Gas mark 4 for 10–15 minutes until piping hot throughout. Leave to cool before serving.

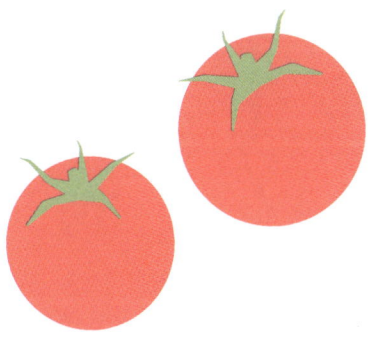

SAUCY DISHES: curries, pasta sauces and stews

Freezing:
Let the food cool thoroughly, then place in an airtight container in the freezer for up to 3 months.

Defrosting:
Defrost fully overnight in the fridge.

Reheating:
Decant into a saucepan and warm through on a low heat on the hob until piping hot throughout.

RICE-BASED DISHES

Freezing:
Make sure you chill down the food quickly. This is essential with rice. You can do this by removing it from the cooked dish and dividing it into smaller containers less than 10cm (4in) deep. Do not stack the containers as the rice cools; sit them next to one another. Once cooled, place in the freezer for up to 3 months.

Defrosting:
Defrost fully overnight in the fridge.

Reheating:
Place the rice in an ovenproof dish, sprinkle with water and cover tightly with foil. Cook at 180°C/160°C fan/350°F/Gas mark 4 for 25–30 minutes until piping hot throughout.

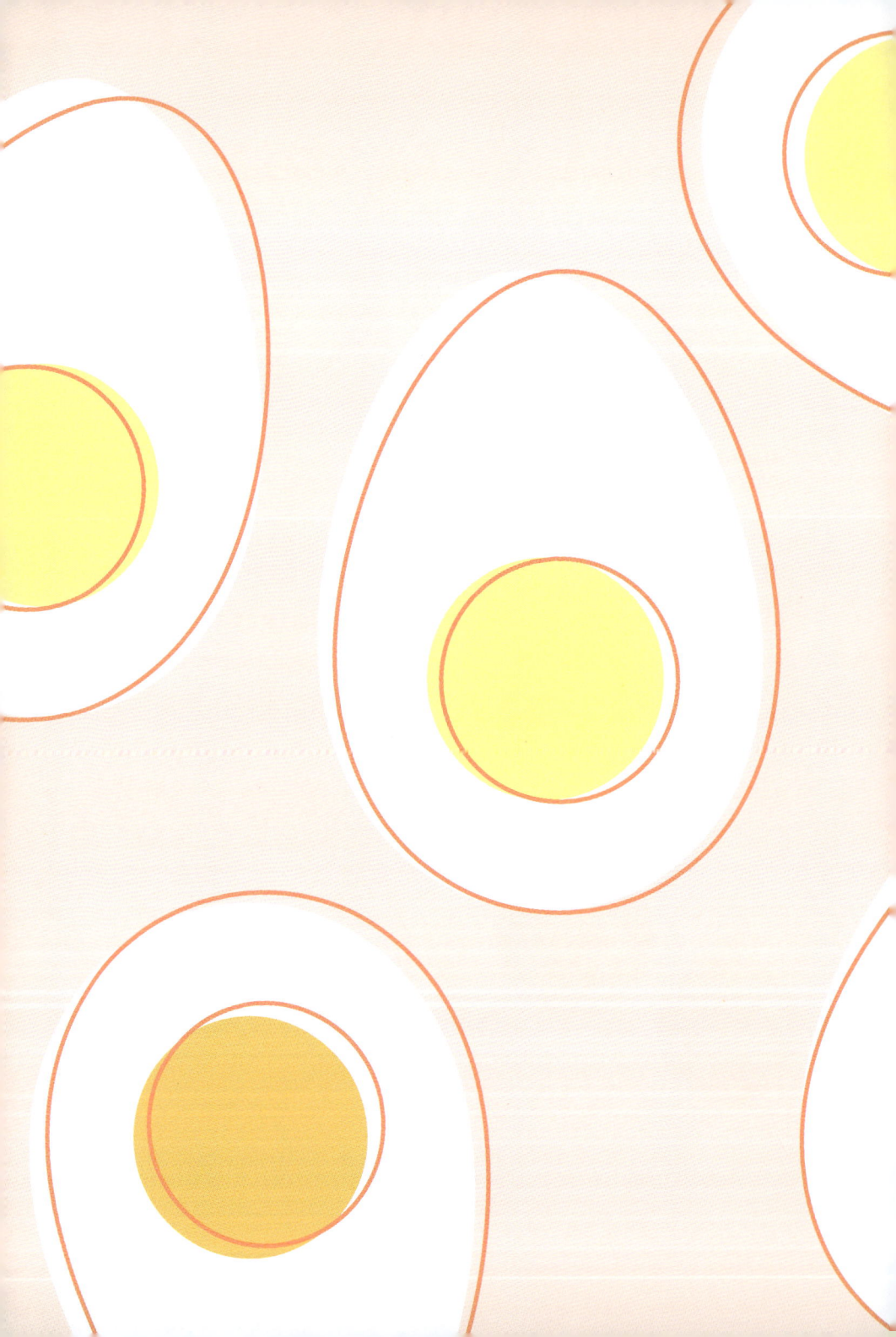

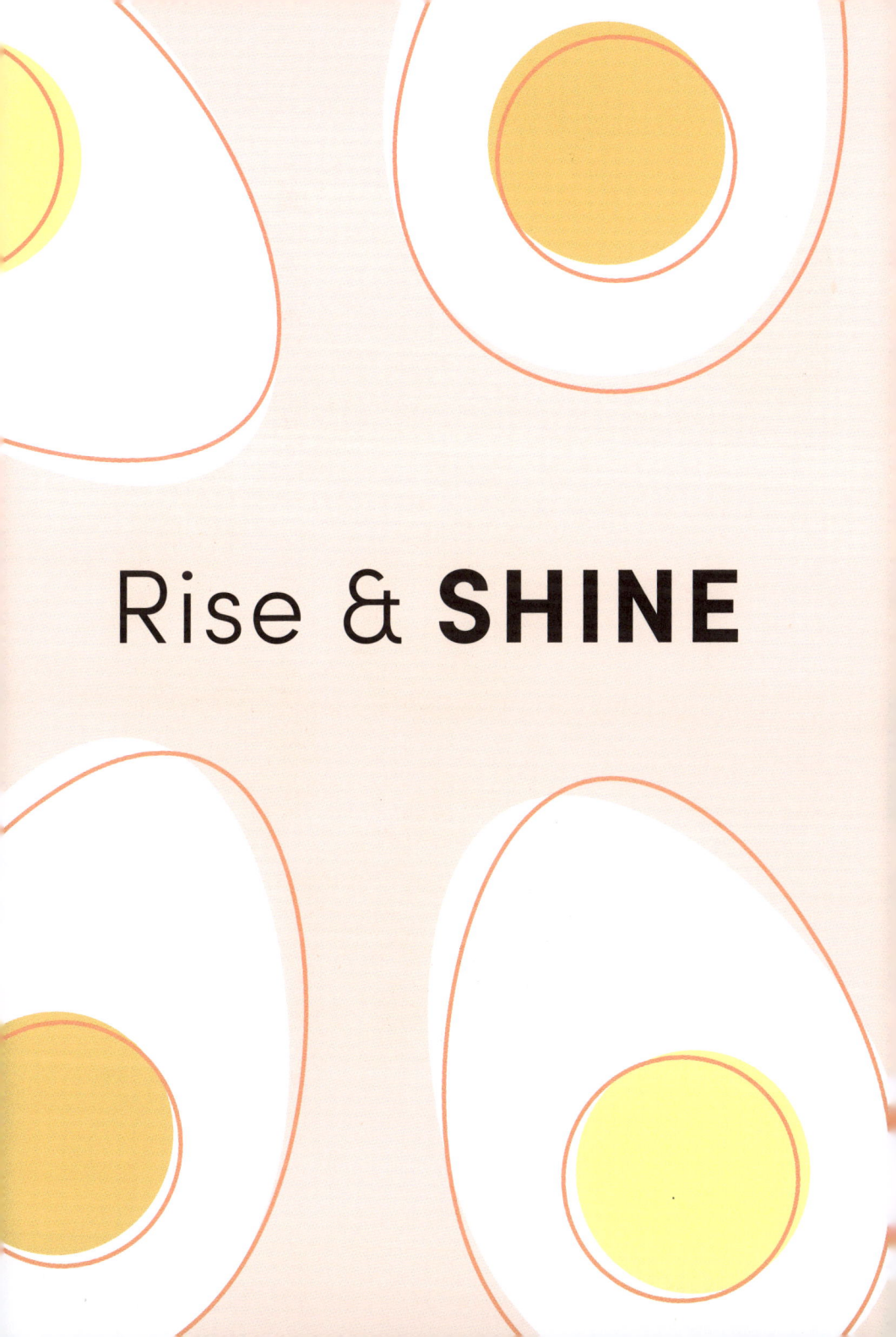

Rise & SHINE

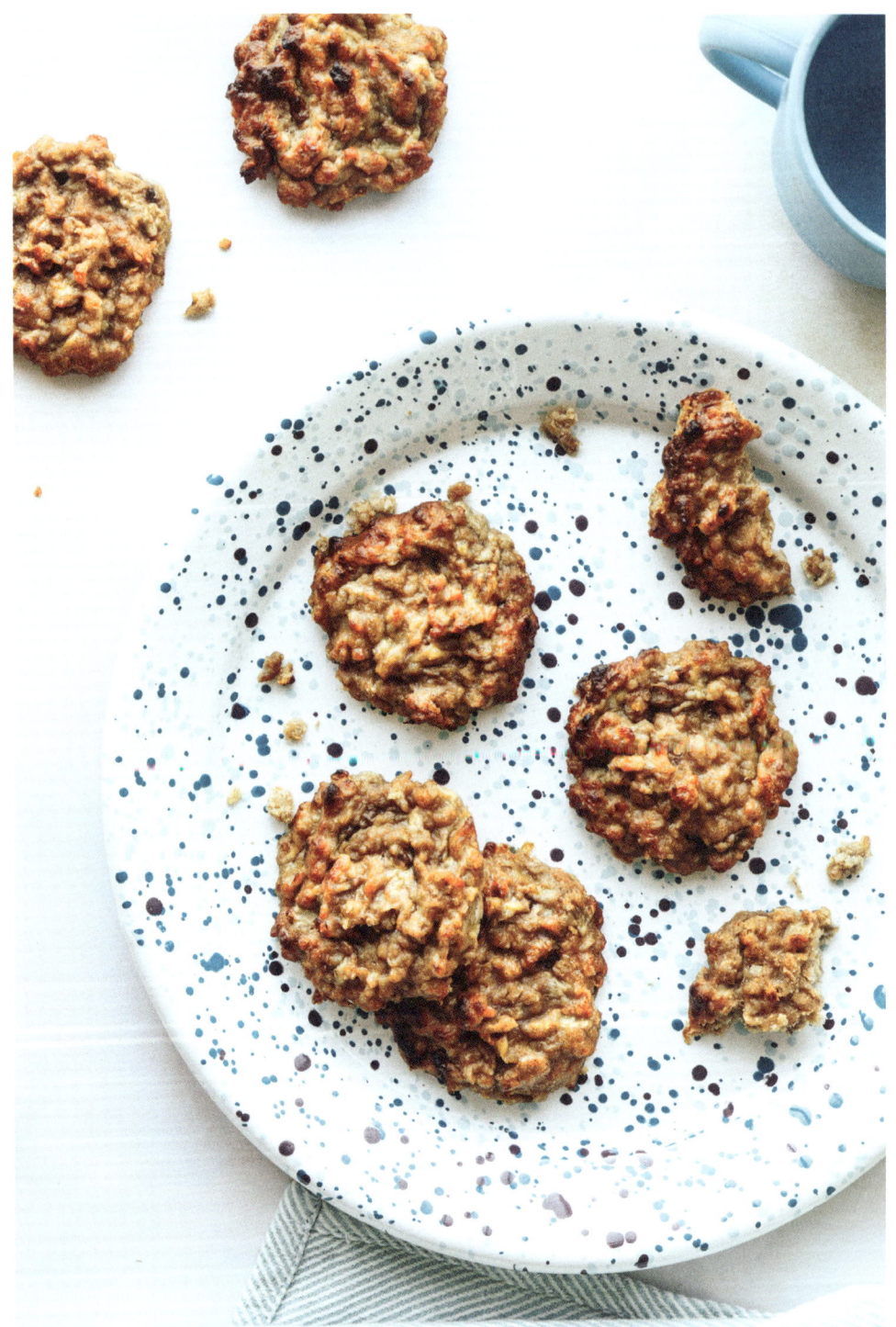

BANANA BREAKFAST BISCUITS

||||||||||||||||||||||||||||||||||||||||||||||||||||||||||||||||||||||||||||||||||||||||||||||||||||||||

Kickstart your little one's day with these nutritious oat-filled banana biscuits. Oats are a treasure trove of vital nutrients, such as manganese, phosphorus, magnesium, iron and essential B vitamins like thiamin and pantothenic acid. Rich in vitamins and healthy fats, these easy yet utterly scrumptious biscuits are sure to 'a-peel' to your baby's tastebuds!

Prep + cook time: **20 mins**

MAKES 8 PORTIONS

3 medium ripe bananas (the riper, the better), mashed
4 tablespoons smooth peanut butter
30g (1oz/⅓ cup) oats

1. Preheat the oven to 200°C/180°C fan/400°F/ Gas mark 6, and grease or line a large baking tray (sheet pan) with baking parchment.
2. Add all the ingredients to a mixing bowl and stir well to combine.
3. Spoon heaped tablespoons of the biscuit mix onto your prepared baking tray, and bake for 15 minutes, or until golden brown. Serve once cooled. Alternatively, air-fry at 160°C/325°F for 12 minutes.

Serving options: Feel free to experiment with these biscuits by adding any optional extras your heart desires, such as finely diced nuts, diced raisins, diced sultanas (golden raisins), diced prunes, diced berries or some low-sugar chocolate chips for a toddler treat when your baby is a little older.

Allergy swaps: For a peanut allergy, swap the peanut butter for sunflower butter or tahini. For a gluten intolerance, use gluten-free oats.

HOMEMADE FRUITY JAM

||||||||||||||||||||||||||||||||||||||||||||||||||||||||||||||||||||||||||||||||||||||||||||||

Who needs shop-bought jam when you can easily make your own healthy version? With only three simple ingredients, this deliciously sweet and sticky jam can be whipped up in under 15 minutes, and is a perfect addition to my Jam and Coconut Pancake Slice (see page 108) and Blueberry Breakfast Scones (see page 115).

Prep + cook time: **15 mins**

MAKES 20 PORTIONS

500g (1lb 2oz/3⅓ cups) any berry variety (strawberries, raspberries, blackberries, etc), pitted cherries or apricots, roughly diced
2 tablespoons maple syrup (optional)
2 tablespoons chia seeds

1. Place the fruit and maple syrup (if using) in a saucepan and heat over a medium heat for 5 minutes, stirring and mashing with a wooden spoon as it cooks down.
2. Lower the heat, then pour in the chia seeds and let the jam simmer for 8 minutes, stirring constantly to ensure it doesn't stick to the pan – as you can imagine, it's very sticky!
3. Remove from the heat and leave the jam to cool and thicken further.
4. Transfer the jam to a sterilized jar or airtight container and store in the refrigerator.

MICROWAVE PORRIDGE FINGERS

||||||||||||||||||||||||||||||||||||||||||||||||||||||||||||||||||||||||||||||||||||||||||||||||||||||||||

This is the ultimate stress- and hassle-free breakfast! The method for these fingers is as easy as 1-2-3: combine the ingredients in an airtight container, flatten the mixture with a spoon, then let the microwave work its magic. And voila! You've just crafted the perfect porridge fingers for your little one.

Prep + cook time: **7 mins**

MAKES 8 PORTIONS

3 tablespoons oats
3 tablespoons whole
   (full-fat) milk
½ teaspoon ground
   cinnamon

1. Add the ingredients to a microwave-safe rectangular airtight container and mix well.
2. Press and flatten the mixture into the base of the container using the back of a spoon.
3. Place the container into the microwave and cook for 2 minutes on high (800W).
4. Slice into fingers and serve once cooled.

   Allergy swaps: For a dairy allergy, swap the milk for soya, oat, coconut, breast or formula milk. For a gluten intolerance, use gluten-free oats.

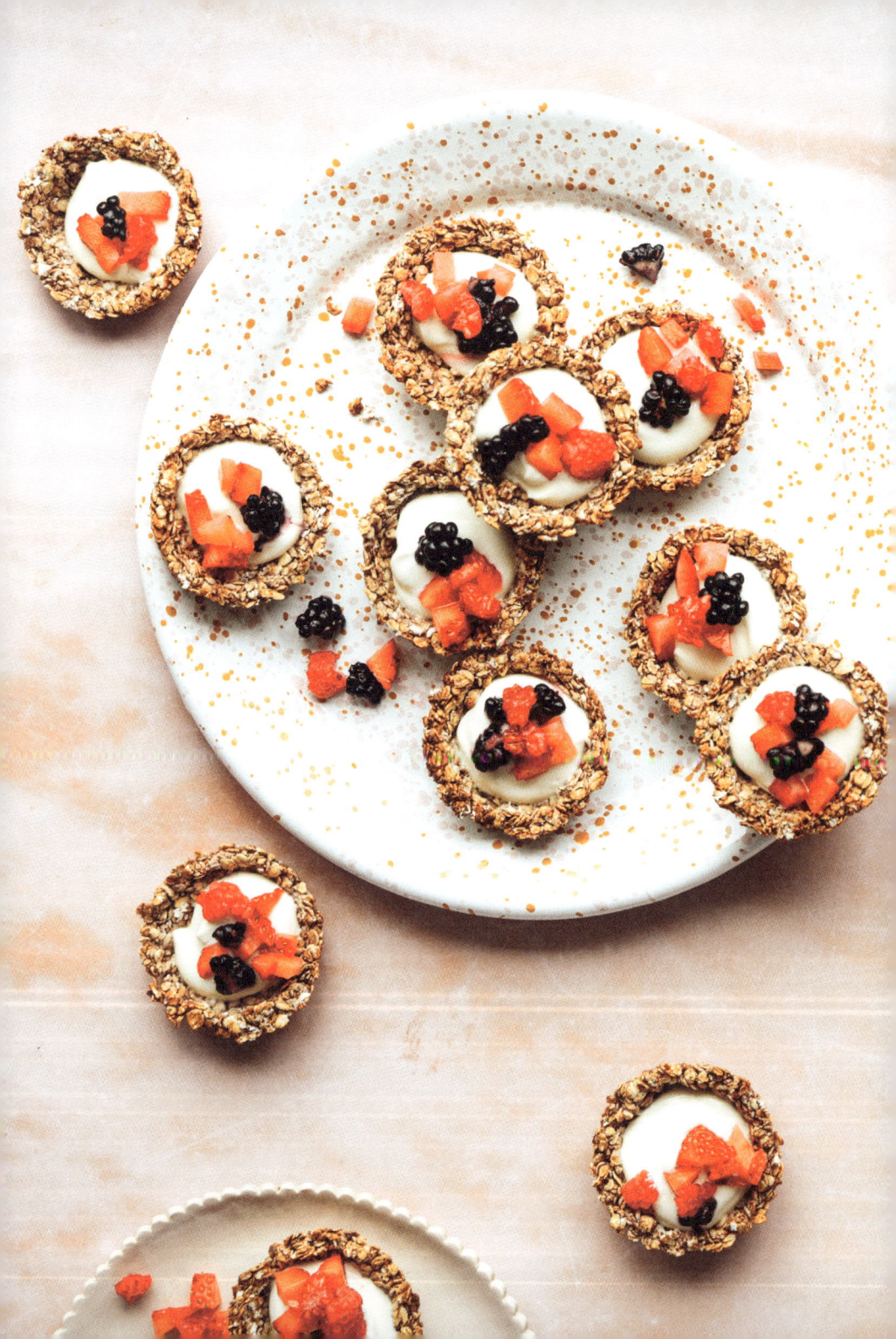

BERRY OAT YOGHURT CUPS

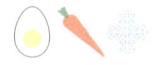

||||||||||||||||||||||||||||||||||||||||||||||||||||||||||||||||||||||||||||||||||||||||

Indulge in these clever yoghurt-filled oat cups that are packed with goodness! Oats offer a wealth of nutrition, with their abundance of vitamins, minerals and fibre, while yoghurt brings essential proteins and calcium, aiding your baby's growth.

Prep + cook time: **20 mins**

MAKES 12 PORTIONS

180g (6½oz/2 cups) oats
1 x 100g (3½oz/scant
    ½ cup) berry fruit purée
    pouch or Pink Purée
    Cubes (see page 188)
2 tablespoons maple
    syrup (optional)
1 teaspoon ground
    cinnamon
12 tablespoons full-fat
    natural yoghurt
75g (2¾oz/½ cup) mixed
    berries, finely chopped

1. Preheat the oven to 200°C/180°C fan/400°F/ Gas mark 6, and grease a 12-hole muffin tray or line with muffin cases.
2. Pour the oats, fruit purée, maple syrup (if using) and cinnamon into a bowl and stir well to combine.
3. Add 1 heaped tablespoon of the mix into each muffin cup, using your thumb to press and pack the oat mixture into the sides and base of each cup.
4. Place the muffin tray into the oven to bake for 12–15 minutes until golden. Alternatively, air-fry at 160°C/325°F for 12 minutes.
5. Once cooked, allow the cups to cool before carefully removing them from the tray. The longer you leave the cups to cool and firm up, the easier it will be to remove them.
6. Fill each cup with a tablespoon of yoghurt and top with a sprinkling of chopped berries. If you plan to freeze the cups, do so before adding the yoghurt and fruit topping.

Allergy swaps: For a dairy allergy, swap the yoghurt for a soya, coconut or oat alternative. For a gluten intolerance, use gluten-free oats.

APRICOT AND VANILLA SWIRL OVERNIGHT OATS

||||||||||||||||||||||||||||||||||||||||||||||||||||||||||||||||||||||||||||||||||||||||||||||||||||

Rise and shine! Whip up these creamy overnight oats before you go to bed for a hearty yet deliciously effortless breakfast the following day.

Prep time: **5 mins, plus overnight resting time**

MAKES 3 PORTIONS

250ml (8½fl oz/1 cup) whole (full-fat) milk

60ml (2fl oz/¼ cup) full-fat natural yoghurt

2½ tablespoons Homemade Fruity Jam made with apricot (see page 100) or use shop-bought low-sugar apricot jam (optional)

½ teaspoon vanilla extract

110g (4oz/1¼ cups) oats

1 tablespoon ground flaxseed (optional)

85g (3oz/½ cup) strawberries, finely diced

1. Place all the ingredients into an airtight container and stir until well combined.
2. Place the container into the refrigerator overnight (for at least 8 hours).
3. Serve, and enjoy!

Serving options: The oats can be served cold, as per the recipe, or you can warm them in the microwave on high (800W) for 30–60 seconds. If your baby doesn't like lumpy textures, you can blend the oats into a smooth porridge.

Allergy swaps: For a dairy allergy, swap the milk for soya, oat, coconut, breast or formula milk, and swap the yoghurt for a soya, coconut or oat alternative. For a gluten intolerance, use gluten-free oats.

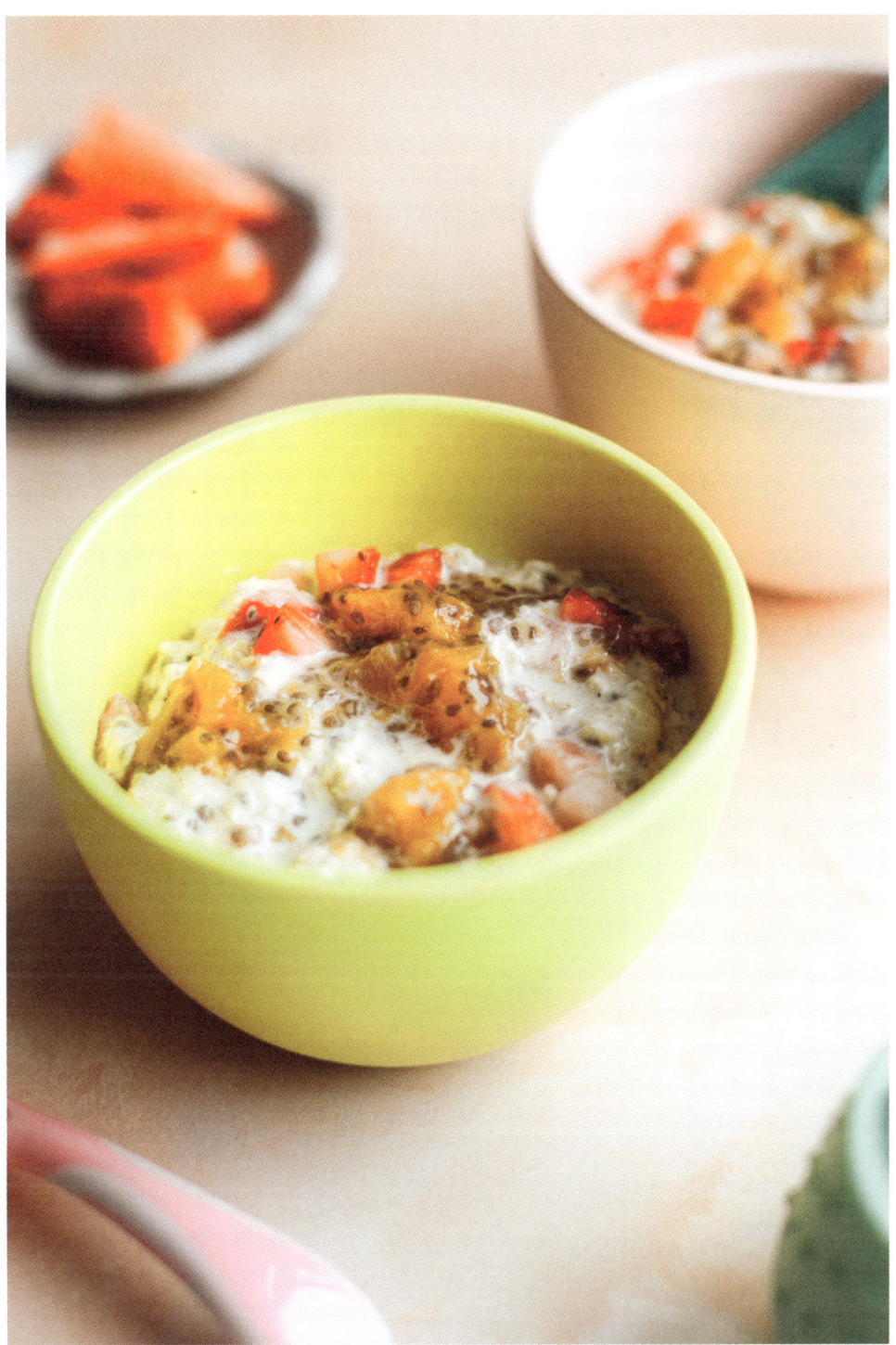

MAKE-AHEAD 5-MINUTE BANANABIX PUDDING

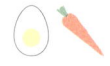

||||||||||||||||||||||||||||||||||||||||||||||||||||||||||||||||||||||||||||||||||||||||||||||||||

Perfectly balanced with the goodness of Weetabix, the creaminess of milk and the natural sweetness of banana, this pudding is a delightful, wholesome introduction to textures for your little one. And it's as easy as it is delicious – just assemble it the evening before, ready for breakfast the following day.

Prep: **5 mins, plus overnight resting time**

MAKES 1 PORTION

2 Weetabix biscuits
125ml (4¼fl oz/½ cup) whole (full-fat) milk
1 tablespoon smooth peanut butter
1 medium banana, mashed
150ml (5fl oz/⅔ cup) full-fat natural yoghurt

1. Crush the Weetabix into the bottom of one of your baby's breakfast bowls.
2. Pour the milk over the Weetabix and stir it through. Once the milk is absorbed, pack the Weetabix down with the back of a spoon to create a 'base'.
3. Smooth the peanut butter over the Weetabix base.
4. In a small bowl, mix the mashed banana with the yoghurt. Once combined, spoon this over the peanut butter.
5. Cover, and place the pudding into the refrigerator overnight (or for at least 4 hours), ready for breakfast the next day.

Allergy swaps: For a dairy allergy, swap the milk for soya, oat, coconut, breast or formula milk, and swap the yoghurt for a soya, coconut or oat alternative. For a peanut allergy, swap the peanut butter for sunflower butter or tahini. For a gluten intolerance, swap the Weetabix for a gluten-free variety.

BAKED FRENCH TOAST

There's no more slaving over a hot stove with this mouthwatering French toast. It's less hands-on than the traditional recipe, making it perfect for busy parents whose hands are needed for spinning many other plates!

Prep + cook time: **18 mins**

MAKES 5 PORTIONS

3 medium eggs
125ml (4¼fl oz/½ cup)
   whole (full-fat) milk
1 tablespoon maple syrup
   (optional)
5 slices white bread

1. Preheat the oven to 200°C/180°C fan/400°F/ Gas mark 6, and grease or line a large baking tray (sheet pan) with baking parchment.
2. Crack the eggs into a shallow-rimmed bowl, then pour in the milk and maple syrup (if using) and whisk well to combine.
3. Carefully dip each bread slice into the egg mix for about 30 seconds each side, then place the slices onto the prepared baking tray.
4. Bake the toast for 10–12 minutes until golden brown and slightly crisp. Serve once cooled. Alternatively, air-fry at 160°C/325°F for 8–10 minutes.

Allergy swaps: For a dairy allergy, swap the milk for soya, oat, coconut, breast or formula milk. For an egg allergy, swap the eggs for two small, mashed bananas (please note, this will add a banana flavour to the toast). For a gluten intolerance, swap the bread for a gluten-free variety.

JAM AND COCONUT PANCAKE SLICE

||||||||||||||||||||||||||||||||||||||||||||||||||||||||||||||||||||||||||||||||||||||||

This irresistible recipe is a twist on the traditional jam and coconut tray bake I enjoyed as a kid. They still serve it at my daughter's school, and it is much loved by many of the children! I hope your whole family enjoys this healthier breakfast version, and that it brings back some fond memories as you enjoy a slice with your baby.

Prep + cook time: **20 mins**

MAKES 8 PORTIONS

375g (13oz/3 cups)
self-raising
(self-rising) flour
3 medium eggs
500ml (17fl oz/2 cups)
whole (full-fat) milk
3 tablespoons Homemade
Fruit Jam (see page
100) or use shop-
bought low-sugar jam
2 tablespoons desiccated
(dried shredded)
coconut

See image overleaf

1. Preheat the oven to 200°C/180°C fan/400°F/ Gas mark 6, and grease or line a rimmed baking tray (sheet pan), approximately 36 x 27cm (14 x 10½in), with baking parchment.
2. Add the flour, eggs and milk to a food processor and blend to form a smooth batter.
3. Pour the batter into the prepared baking tray and smooth out with the back of a spoon.
4. Place the tray into the oven to bake for 15 minutes, or until golden and cooked through.
5. Allow the sheet pancake to cool slightly, then spread over the jam and sprinkle with the coconut before serving. If freezing, do so before adding the jam and coconut topping.

Allergy swaps: Swap the milk for soya, oat, coconut, breast or formula milk. For an egg allergy, swap the eggs for 2 small mashed bananas (this will add a banana flavour to the pancake slice). For a coconut allergy, swap the coconut for finely diced macadamia nuts, or omit completely. For a gluten intolerance, swap the flour for a gluten-free variety.

STRAWBERRY AND MASCARPONE PANCAKES

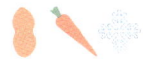

||||||||||||||||||||||||||||||||||||||||||||||||||||||||||||||||||||||||||||||||||||||||||||||||

These thick, fluffy pancakes are a breakfast delight – and as an added bonus, they also freeze beautifully! Bursting with calcium and protein, they are an excellent choice for a nutritious and satisfying start to the morning.

Prep + cook time: **20 mins**

MAKES 8 PORTIONS

120g (4¼oz/1 cup)
   self-raising
   (self-rising) flour
3 large eggs
250g (9oz/1 cup)
   mascarpone cheese
1 teaspoon vanilla extract
85g (3oz/½ cup)
   strawberries, hulled and
   finely diced
1 teaspoon vegetable oil,
   plus extra as needed

See image overleaf

1. Pour the flour into a mixing bowl.
2. Crack the eggs into a jug (pitcher), then whisk together with the mascarpone cheese and vanilla extract.
3. Slowly add the wet ingredients to the flour, whisking until there are no lumps and you have a smooth, thick batter.
4. Fold through the finely diced strawberries.
5. In a frying pan (skillet), heat the oil over a medium heat, then add 2 tablespoons of batter per pancake.
6. Fry the pancakes for 2 minutes until bubbles start to form on top, then flip and fry for a further 2 minutes until golden brown. Repeat with the remaining batter (adding a little more oil if needed). Leave to cool slightly, then serve.

Allergy swaps: For a dairy allergy, swap the mascarpone for a dairy-free soft cream cheese. For an egg allergy, swap the eggs for 3 tablespoons ground flaxseed stirred into 9 tablespoons water. For a gluten intolerance, swap the flour for a gluten-free variety.

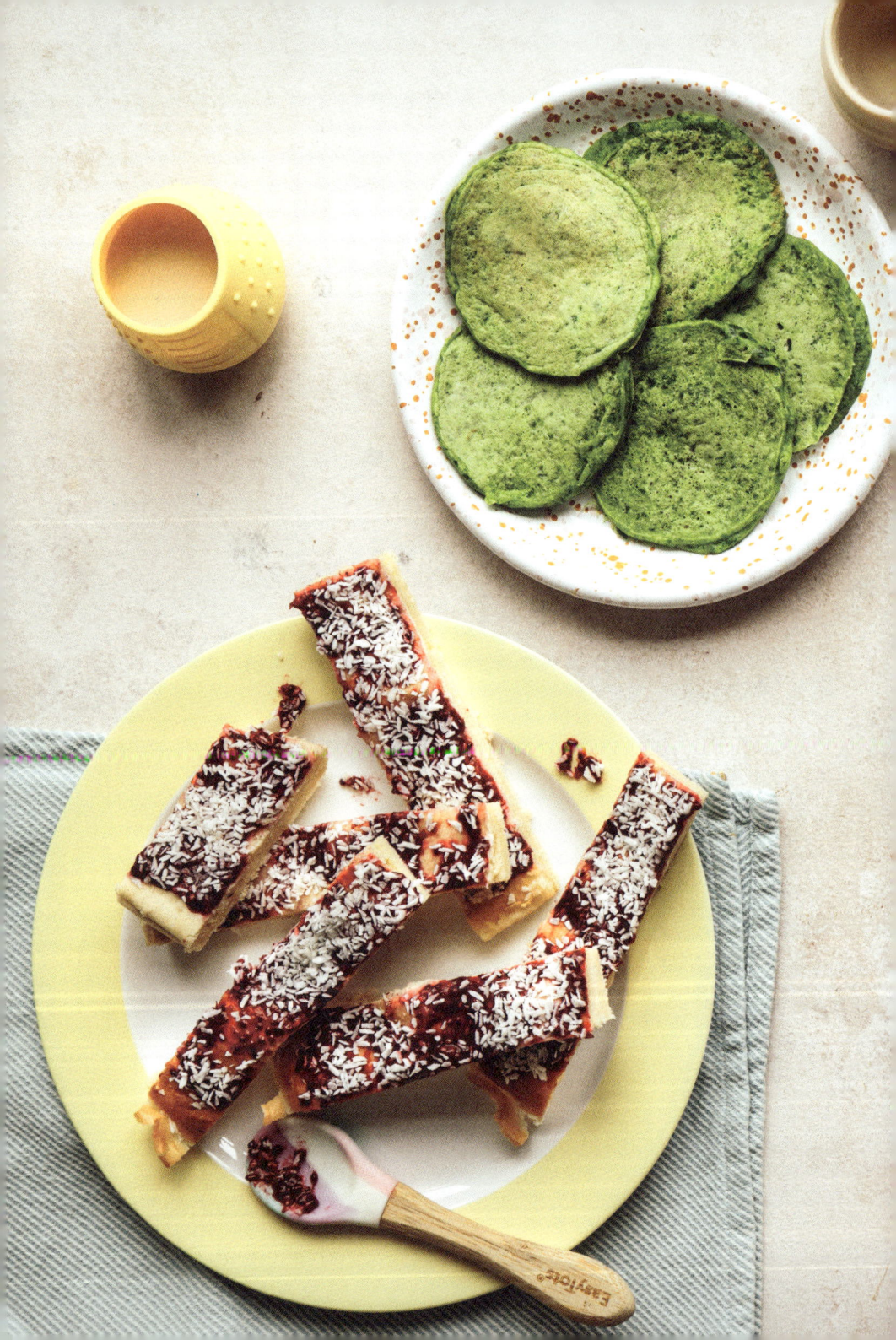

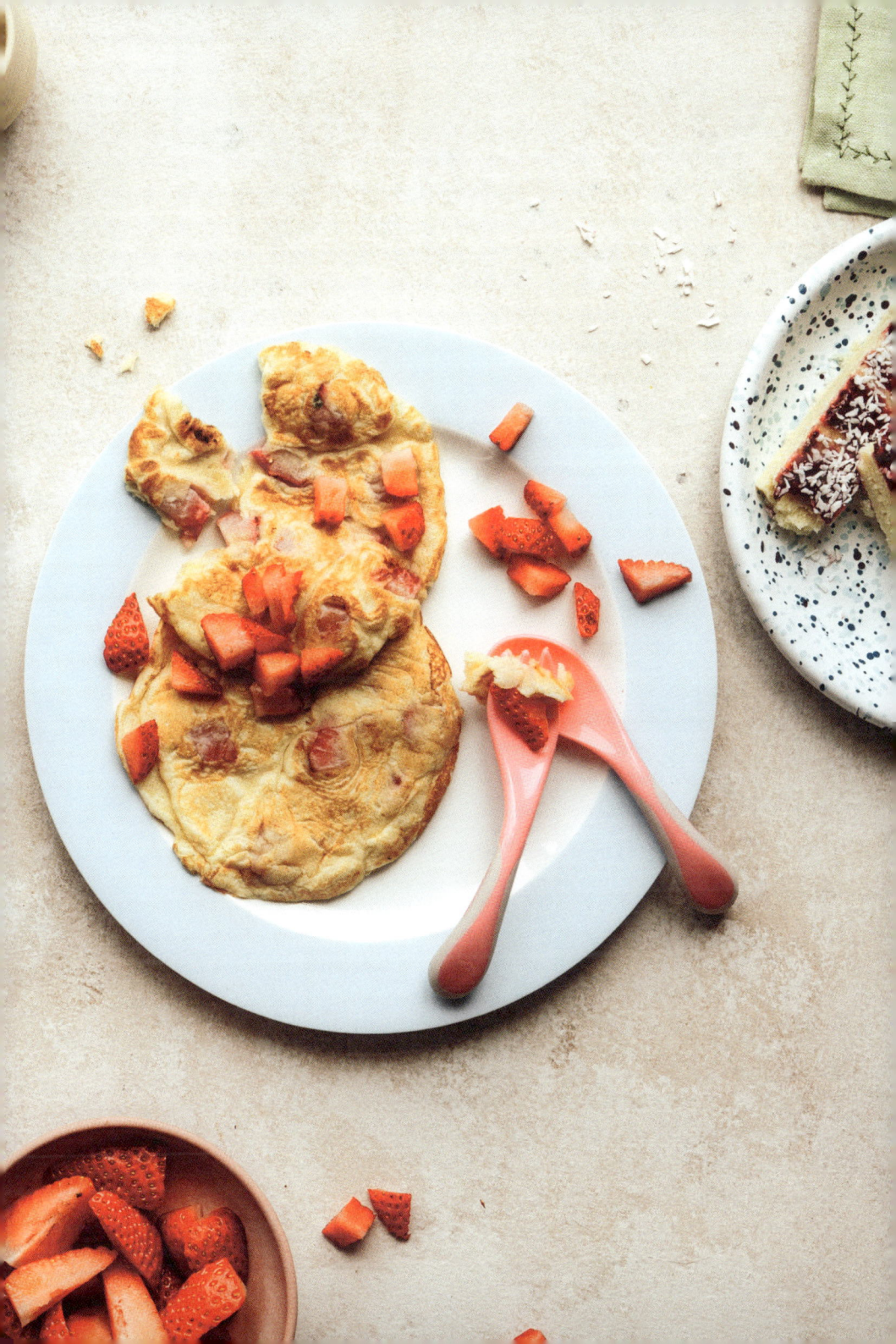

HULK PANCAKES

These scrumptious super-hero pancakes are loaded with iron-rich spinach, as well as protein, making a fun and wholesome breakfast option for your little champion.

Prep + cook time: **20 mins**

MAKES 14-16 PORTIONS

120g (4¼oz/1 cup)
self-raising
(self-rising) flour
90g (3oz/3 cups) spinach
1 medium egg
250ml (8½fl oz/1 cup)
whole (full-fat) milk
1 teaspoon vegetable oil

1. Add all the ingredients, except the oil, into a blender or food processor and blend until smooth.
2. In a frying pan (skillet), heat the oil over a medium heat, then add 2 tablespoons of batter per pancake – fry each pancake for 2 minutes on each side, or until the rich green colour takes on a slightly golden tone. Leave to cool slightly, then serve.

Allergy swaps: For a dairy allergy, swap the milk for soya, oat, coconut, breast or formula milk. For an egg allergy, swap the egg for 1 small mashed banana (please note, this will add a banana flavour to the pancakes). For a gluten intolerance, swap the flour for a gluten-free variety.

NOTE

You will know when the pancakes are ready to flip as bubbles will form on the top; as soon as you see three or more bubbles, getting flipping!

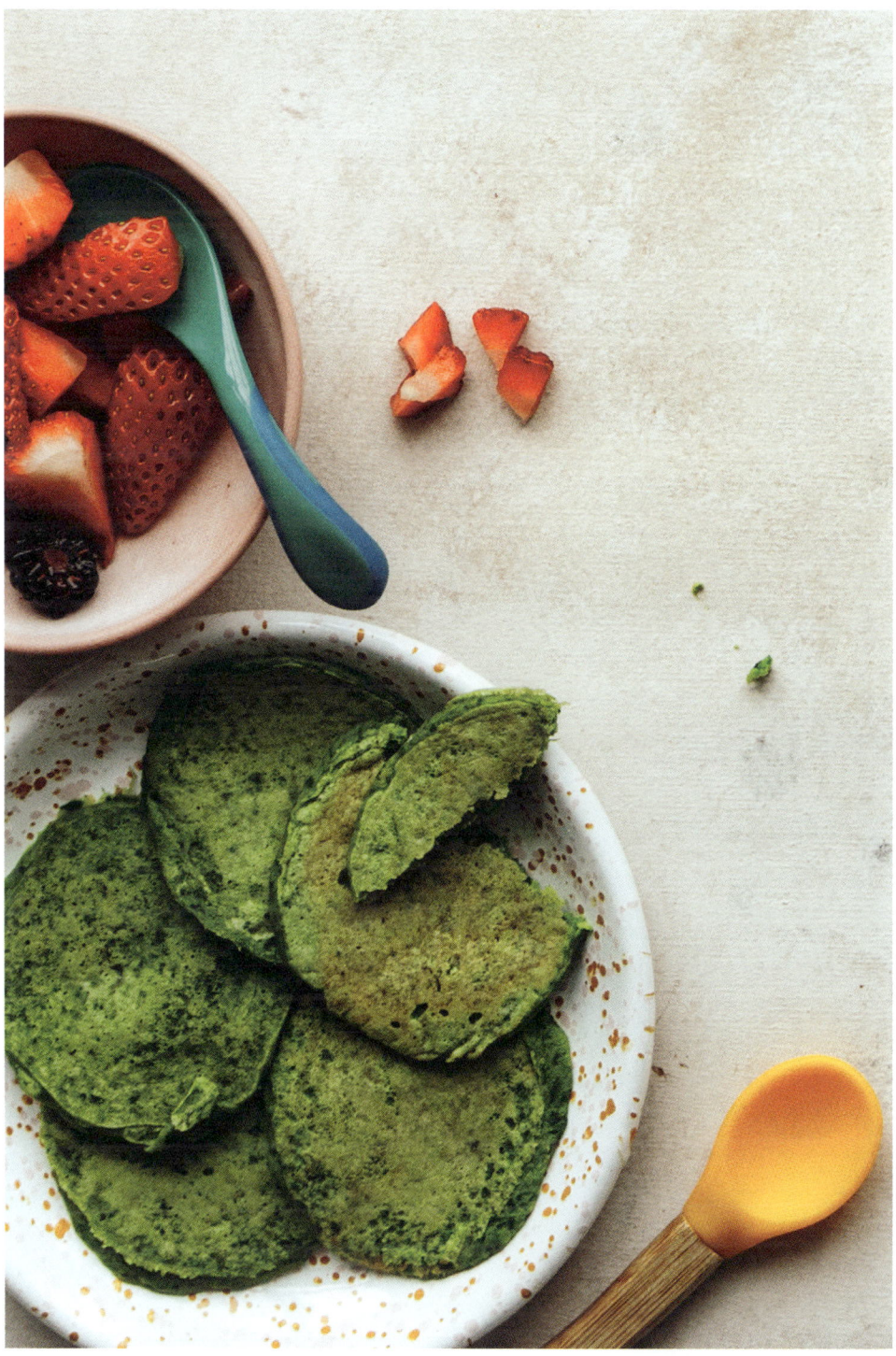

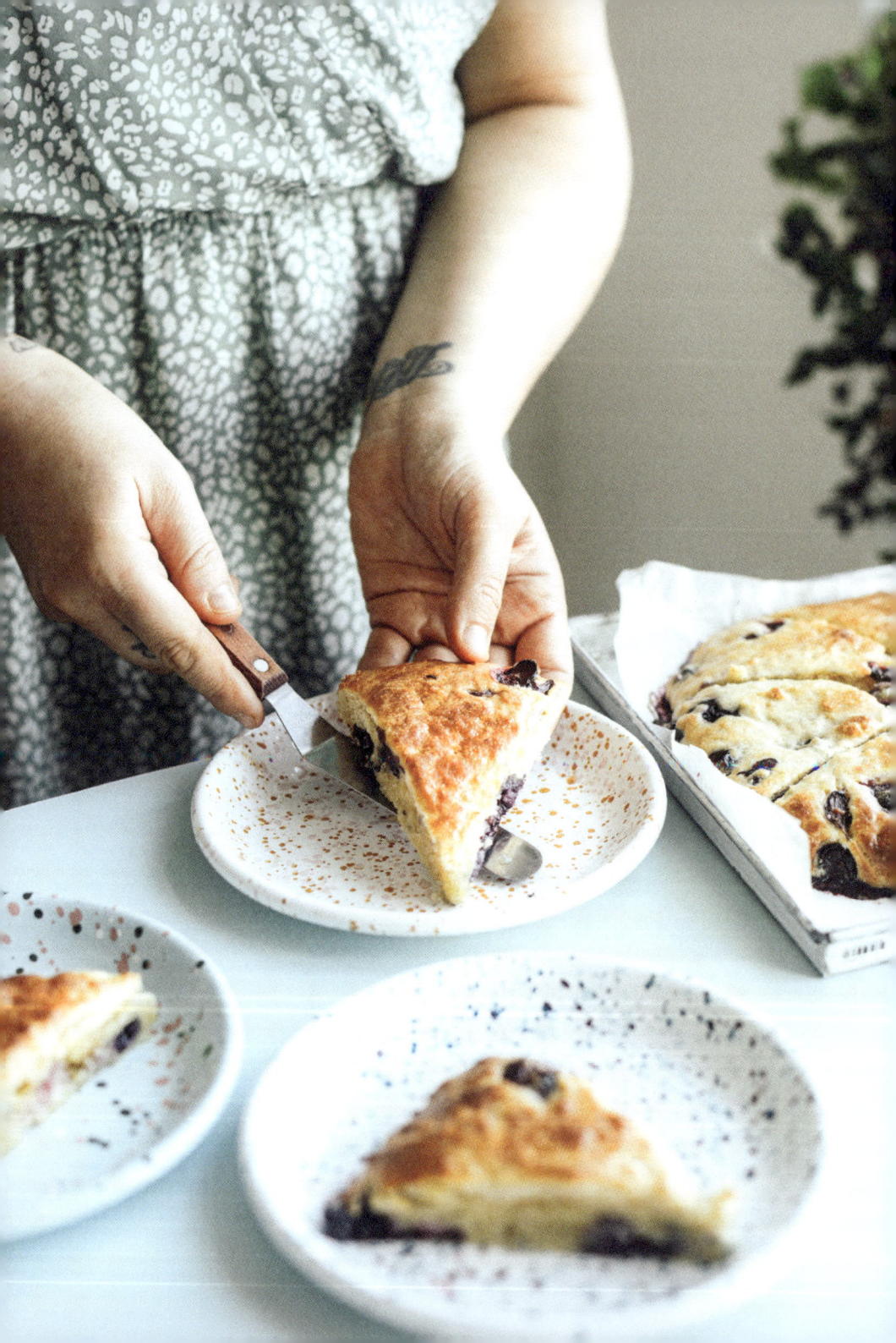

BLUEBERRY BREAKFAST SCONES

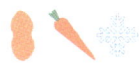

I have to hide these scones from my husband, Steve, as he will eat them all before my children get a look in! Unlike traditional English scones made with butter, these are made with cream, which gives them an irresistibly soft consistency.

Prep + cook time: **20 mins**

MAKES 8 PORTIONS

240g (8½oz/2 cups) self-raising (self-rising) flour
60ml (2fl oz/¼ cup) maple syrup or fruit purée
250ml (8½fl oz/1 cup) double (heavy) cream
1 medium egg
95g (3½oz/½ cup) blueberries, sliced in half through the stem
2 teaspoons whole (full-fat) milk

1. Preheat the oven to 220°C/200°C fan/425°F/ Gas mark 7, and grease or line a large baking tray (sheet pan) with baking parchment.
2. Add the flour to a mixing bowl.
3. Pour the maple syrup, cream and egg into a jug and whisk to combine.
4. Slowly pour the wet mix into the dry and start to combine with a wooden spoon.
5. Add the blueberries, then bring together with your hands to form a thick dough.
6. Place the dough onto a lightly floured surface and roll it into a large circle, about 2cm (¾in) in thickness.
7. Slice the dough into 8 triangles (like a pizza), then place the triangles onto the prepared baking tray.
8. Brush the scones with milk and bake for about 15 minutes, or until golden. Leave to cool, then serve. Alternatively, air-fry at 180°C/350°F for 12 minutes.

Allergy swaps: Swap the milk for soya, oat, coconut, breast or formula milk, and use a dairy-free cream alternative of your choice. Swap the egg for 1 tablespoon ground flaxseed stirred into 3 tablespoons water. Swap the flour for gluten-free.

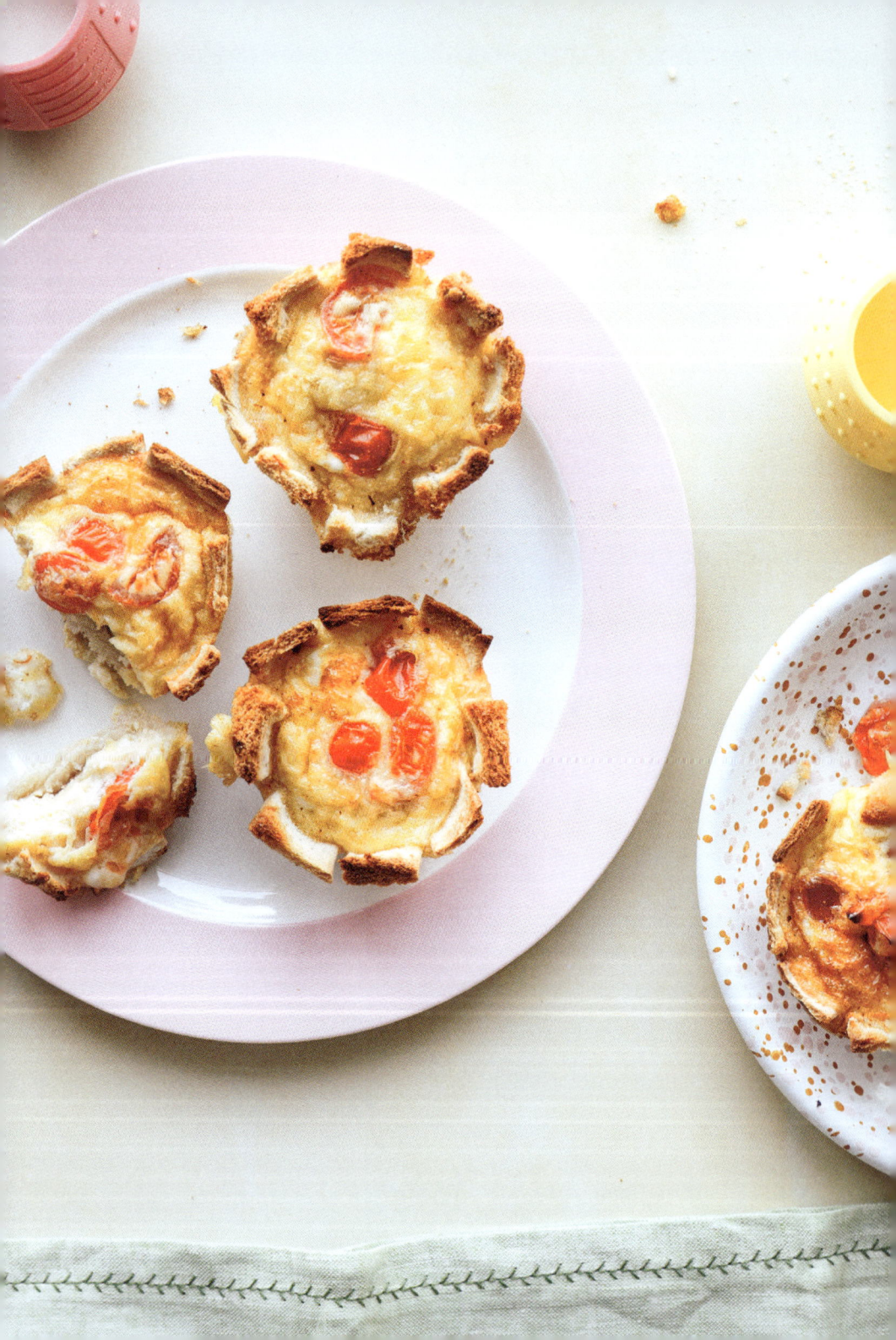

TOASTED EGG CUPS

||||||||||||||||||||||||||||||||||||||||||||||||||||||||||||||||||||||||||||||||||||||

These easy, protein-packed egg cups are quick to whip up and easy for little hands to hold, as the toasted base makes them less slippery than traditional egg muffin cup recipes. You can customize this recipe with different fillings as an easy way to add variety to your baby's diet – try finely diced spinach or peppers, shredded or finely chopped chicken, or leftover vegetables.

Prep + cook time: **20 mins**

MAKES 6 PORTIONS

6 slices white bread, crusts removed
5 medium eggs
110g (4oz/½ cup) grated Cheddar cheese
50g (1¾oz/⅓ cup) cherry tomatoes, sliced into quarters

1. Preheat the oven to 200°C/180°C fan/400°F/ Gas mark 6, and grease 6 holes of a 12-hole muffin tray or line with muffin cases.
2. Using a rolling pin, flatten the bread slices until they are 5mm (¼in) thick.
3. Cut each flattened slice of bread into 4 long batons, then push the 4 batons down into each muffin cup, creating star-shaped cups.
4. Whisk the eggs in a jug, then stir through the cheese and cherry tomatoes.
5. Pour the egg mix into the cups, dividing it evenly between each one.
6. Bake for 15 minutes, then remove from the oven carefully and serve once cooled.

Allergy swaps: For a dairy allergy, swap the cheese for a dairy-free Cheddar. For an egg allergy, use 'vegan' eggs, which are available at most health food stores. For a gluten intolerance, swap the bread for a gluten-free variety.

TOASTED BREAKFAST SANDWICH FIVE WAYS

A toasted breakfast sandwich is quick to prepare and can be adapted to include many different flavour combinations. Here are five of our family favourites, but I encourage you to experiment with other varieties – and for lunch, too.

Prep + cook time: **10 mins**

MAKES 1–2 PORTIONS

2 slices bread
1 teaspoon unsalted
   butter
1 teaspoon vegetable oil

Filling option 1:
2 teaspoons smooth
   peanut butter
1 small banana, mashed

Filling option 2:
1 tablespoon vegan pesto
½ tomato, finely diced
1 handful of grated
   cheese of your choice

1. Butter the slices of bread as if making a sandwich and add your desired fillings.
2. Close the sandwich and heat the oil in a frying pan (skillet) over a low-medium heat.
3. Once hot, add the sandwich and toast for 2–3 minutes on each side until golden brown and crispy.
4. Slice into soldiers and serve once cooled.

Allergy swaps: For a dairy allergy, swap the butter for a dairy-free butter alternative, and swap the cheese for a dairy-free grated or soft cheese. For a peanut allergy, swap the peanut butter for sunflower butter or tahini. For a gluten intolerance, swap the bread for a gluten-free variety.

Filling option 3:
3 tablespoons baked
   beans, mashed
1 handful of grated cheese
   of your choice

Filling option 4:
1 tablespoon cream
   cheese
1 teaspoon low-sugar jam
1 banana, sliced

Filling option 5:
1 tablespoon cream
   cheese
1 small apple or pear,
   peeled and thinly sliced

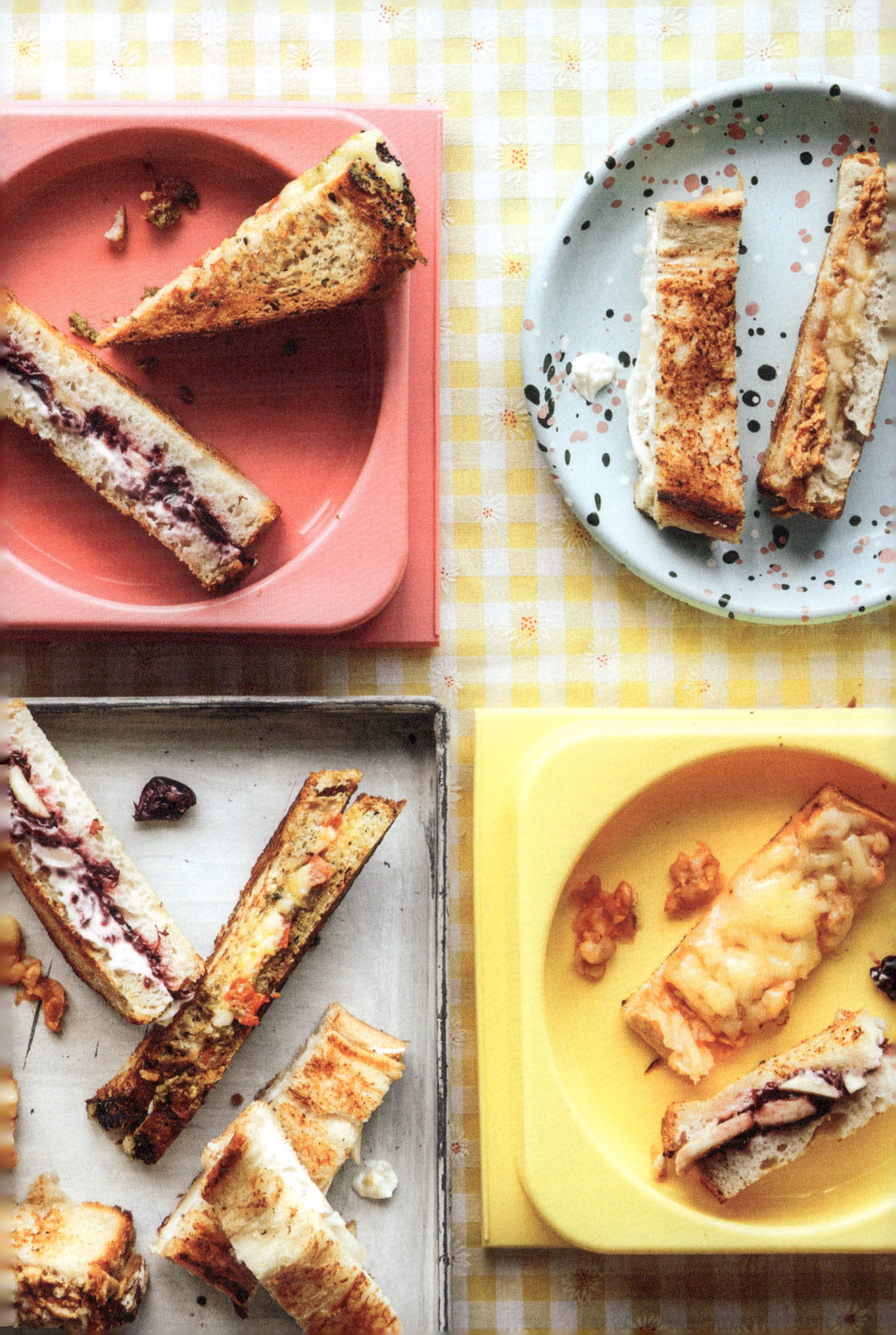

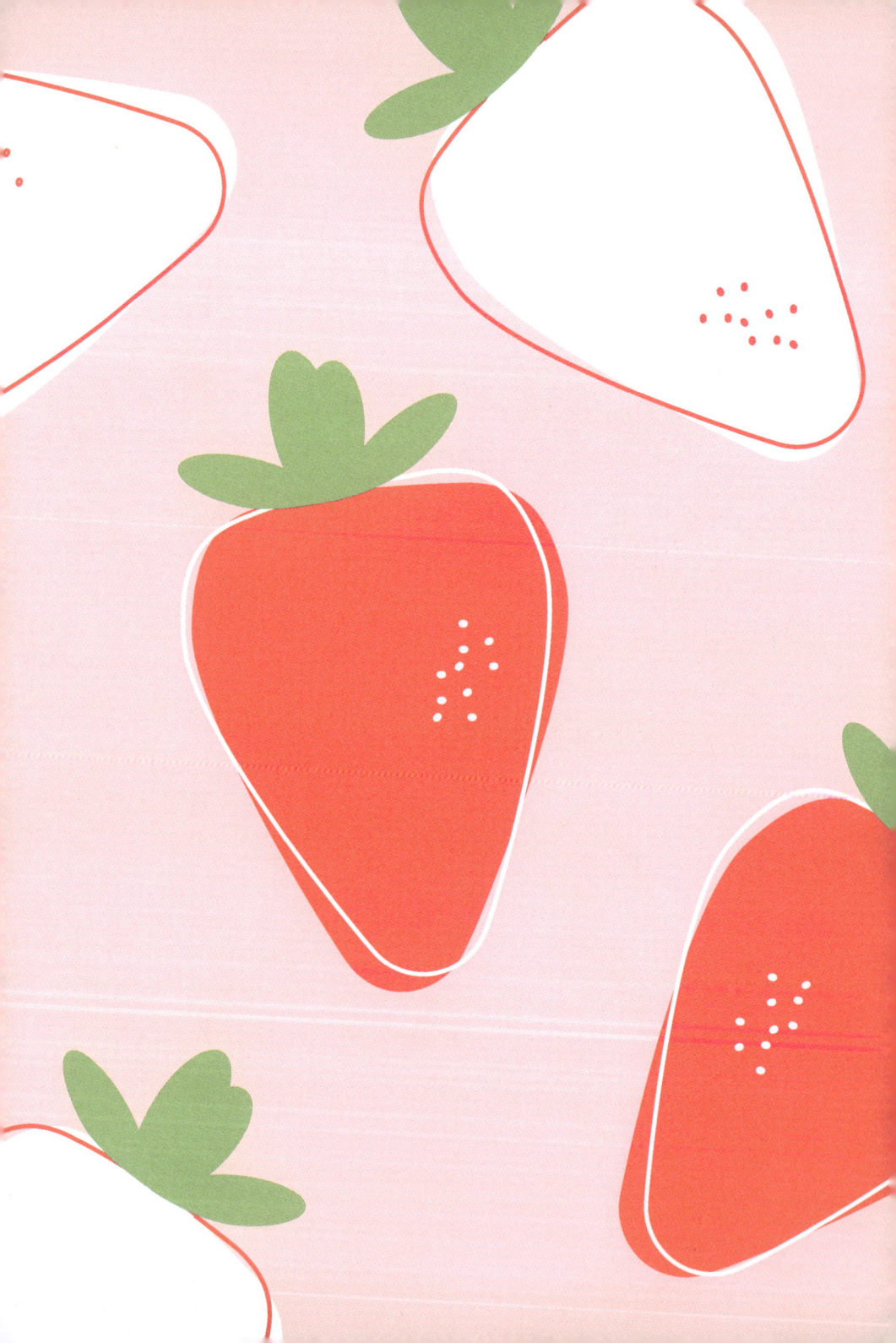

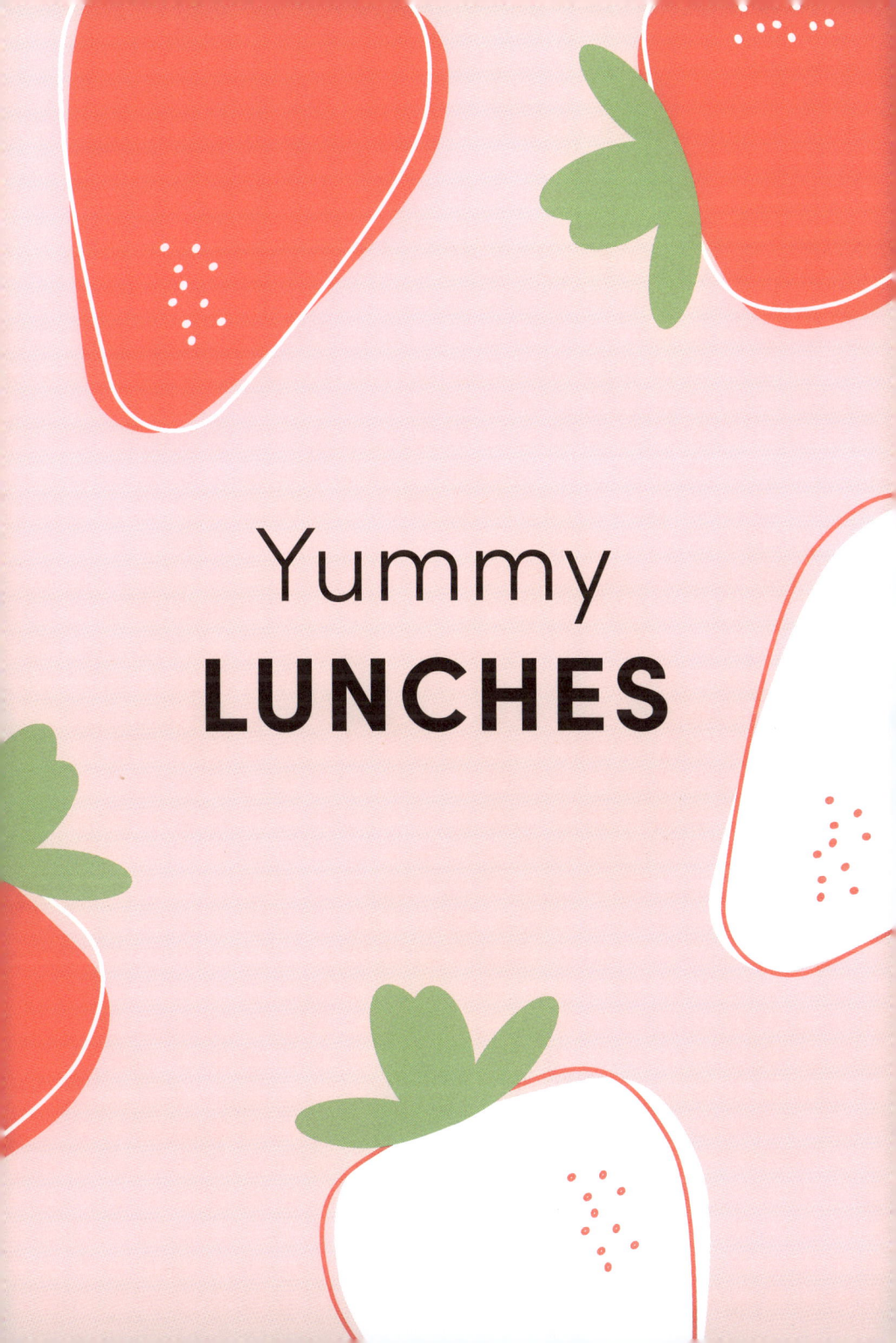

Yummy
LUNCHES

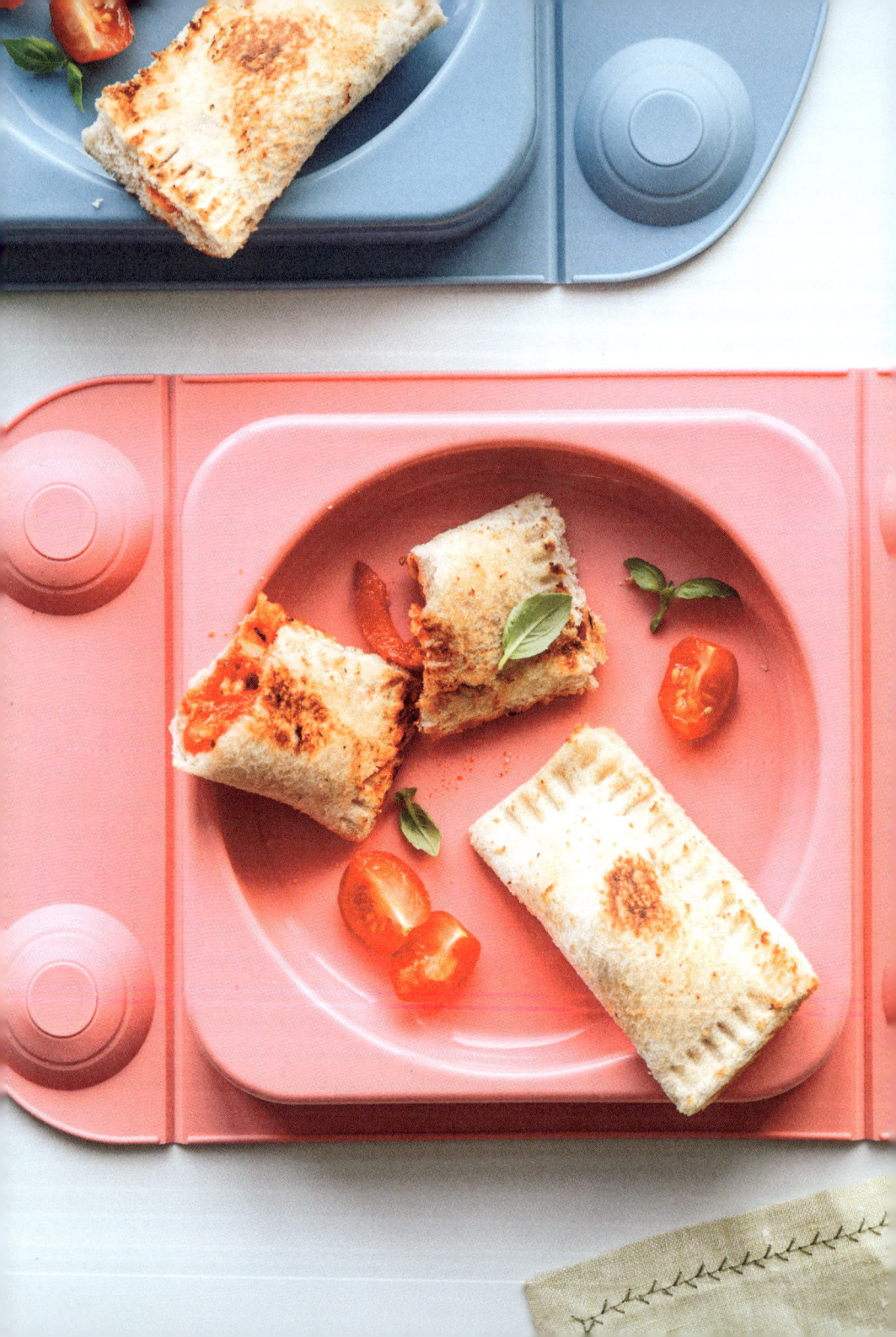

EASY PIZZA POCKETS

|||||||||||||||||||||||||||||||||||||||||||||||||||||||||||||||||||||||||||||||||||||||||||||||||||||||||||||

These pizza pockets are a super-speedy lunch option, bursting with saucy tomato, sweet red pepper and gooey cheese.

Prep + cook time: **20 mins**
Cook time: **12 mins**

MAKES 6 PORTIONS

2 teaspoons vegetable oil
1 small onion, very
   finely diced
1 red (bell) pepper,
   deseeded and thinly
   sliced
½ teaspoon minced garlic
120g (4¼oz/1 cup) grated
   Cheddar cheese
3 tablespoons tomato
   purée (paste)
½ teaspoon dried basil
6 slices white bread,
   crusts removed

1. Heat 1 teaspoon of the vegetable oil in a large frying pan (skillet) over a medium heat, then add the diced onion and sliced pepper and fry for 5 minutes until softened.
2. Turn off the heat and stir through the minced garlic, grated cheese, tomato purée (paste) and basil. Set aside.
3. Using a rolling pin, flatten the bread slices until they are 5mm (¼in) thick.
4. Divide the filling evenly between the 6 slices of bread, spooning it over the bottom half of each slice, leaving a 5mm (¼in) border around the edge.
5. Carefully fold the bread slices to conceal the filling and form 6 rectangular pizza pockets. Seal the sides of the pockets using the back of a fork, creating a crinkle effect.
6. Heat another teaspoon of oil in the frying pan, add the pockets in two batches, and frying each batch for 2–3 minutes on each side until golden and crispy. Serve once cooled.

Allergy swaps: For a dairy allergy, swap the cheese for a dairy-free Cheddar. For a gluten intolerance, swap the bread for a gluten-free variety.

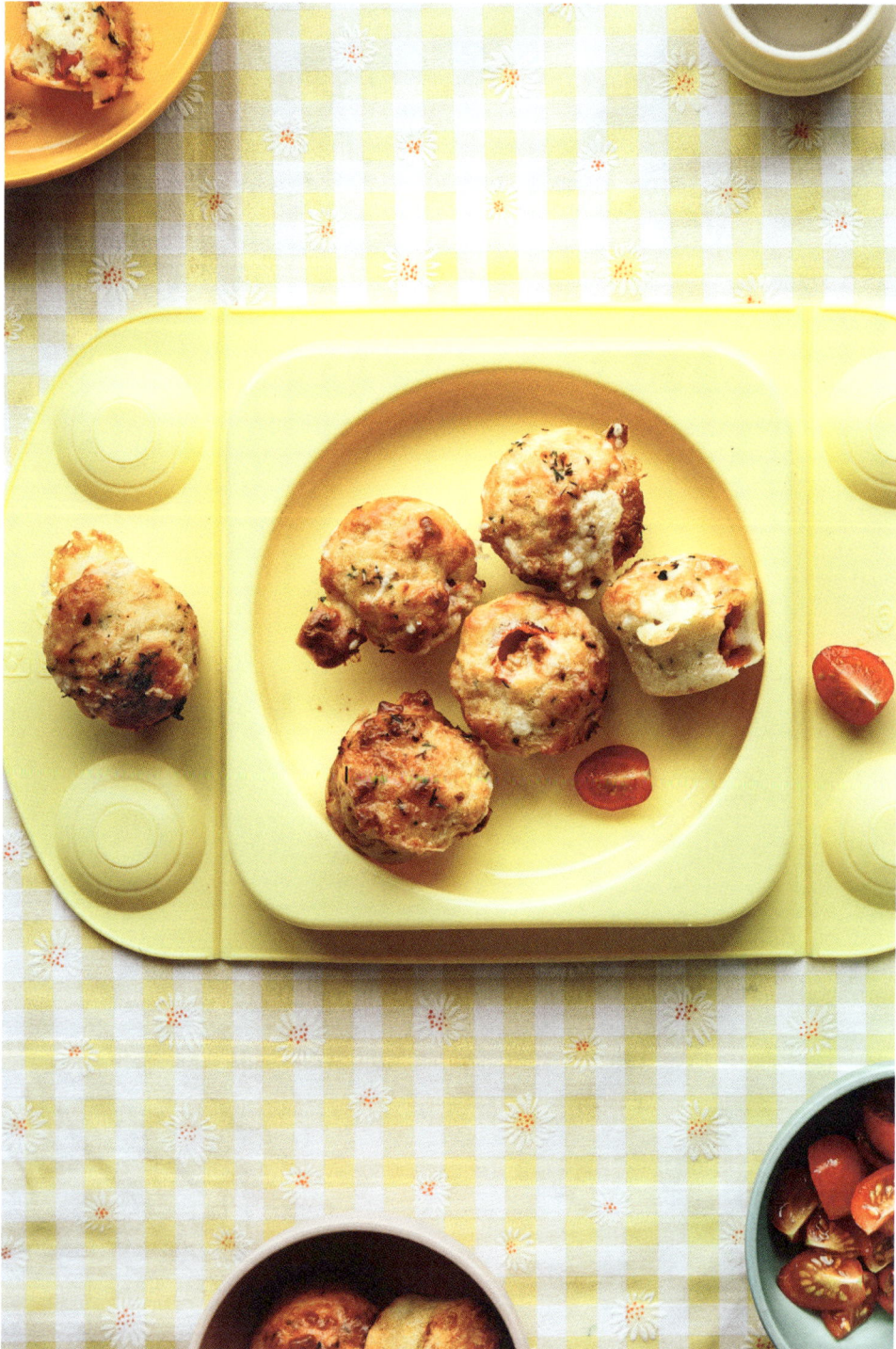

CHEESE AND TOMATO MINI MUFFINS

||||||||||||||||||||||||||||||||||||||||||||||||||||||||||||||||||||||||||||||||||||||||||||||||||||

Tiny hands, big flavours! With just the right blend of wholesome ingredients, these soft cheese and tomato bites are not only irresistibly delicious, but also a wonderfully nourishing lunch option, and will become a family favourite in no time.

Prep + cook time: **20 mins**

MAKES 24 PORTIONS

240g (8½oz/2 cups)
   self-raising
   (self-rising) flour
60ml (2fl oz/¼ cup)
   vegetable oil
125ml (4¼fl oz/½ cup)
   whole (full-fat) milk
3 medium eggs, beaten
1½ teaspoons mixed
   herbs
180g (6½oz/1½ cups)
   grated Cheddar cheese,
   plus extra for sprinkling
150g (5oz/1 cup) cherry
   tomatoes, sliced into
   quarters

1. Preheat the oven to 210°C/190°C fan/425°F/Gas mark 7, and grease a 24-hole mini-muffin tray or line with mini-muffin cases.
2. Place the flour, oil, milk, eggs and mixed herbs into a large mixing bowl and stir to combine.
3. Fold through the cheese and cherry tomatoes.
4. Divide the mixture evenly between the holes of the mini-muffin tray and sprinkle with a little extra cheese.
5. Place the muffins into the oven to bake for 15 minutes, or until golden and a knife comes out clean from the centre. Serve once cooled.

Allergy swaps: For a dairy allergy, swap the milk for soya, oat, coconut, breast or formula milk, and swap the cheese for a dairy-free grated Cheddar. For an egg allergy, swap the eggs for 3 tablespoons ground flaxseed stirred into 9 tablespoons water. For a gluten intolerance, swap the flour for a gluten-free variety.

CURRIED CARROT FRITTERS

||||||||||||||||||||||||||||||||||||||||||||||||||||||||||||||||||||||||||||||||||||||||||||||||||

Introduce your little one to the exciting world of spice with my curried fritters! These baby-led weaning delights are simple to make and bursting with grated carrots and a warm, subtle, spicy flavour.

Prep + cook time: **20 mins**

MAKES 9 PORTIONS

2 medium eggs
60g (2oz/½ cup)
   self-raising
   (self-rising) flour
½ red onion, very finely
   diced
2 small carrots, grated
1 tablespoon mild curry
   powder
1 tablespoon vegetable oil

1. Place all of the ingredients, except the oil, into a large mixing bowl and stir well to combine.
2. Heat the oil in a large frying pan (skillet) over a medium heat.
3. Add heaped tablespoons of the mix into the frying pan, and cook for 2–3 minutes, then flip each one and cook the underside for 2–3 minutes until golden and crispy. Continue until all the mixture has been used. You should be able to fit 3 fritters into a pan at a time, so will need to cook them in 3 batches. Serve once cooled.

Allergy swaps: For an egg allergy, swap the eggs for 2 tablespoons ground flaxseed stirred into 6 tablespoons water. For a gluten intolerance, swap the flour for a gluten-free variety.

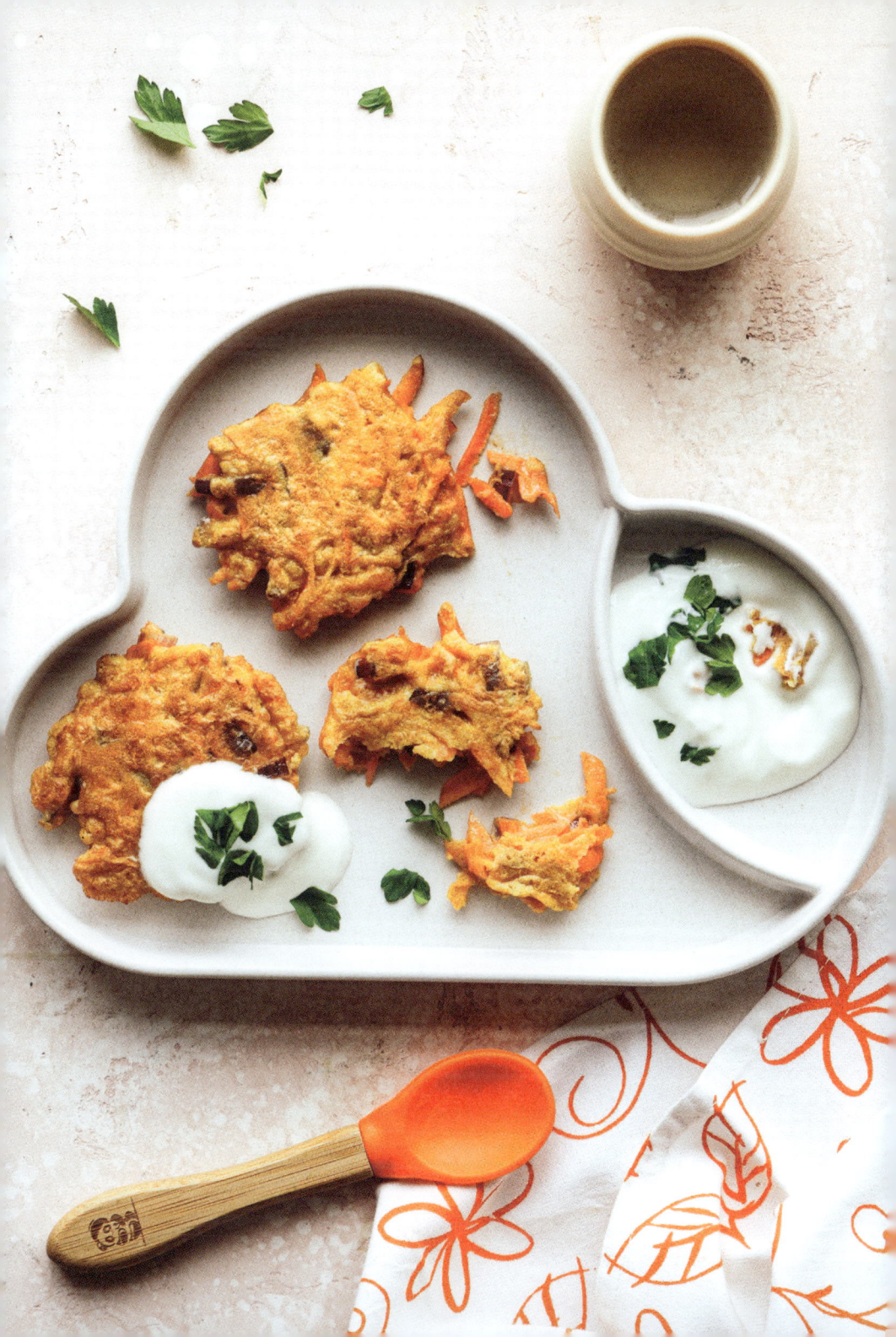

SWEET POTATO MELTS

Get ready to savour the irresistible delight of sweet potato melts – a playful and enticing spin on the classic sandwich melt. The long, finger-sized batons are perfect for tiny hands.

Prep + cook time: **20 mins**

MAKES 4 PORTIONS

1 small sweet potato,
   sliced into 1cm (½in)
   circles
120g (4¼oz/½ cup)
   tomato purée (paste)
2 teaspoons mixed herbs
90g (3oz/¾ cup) grated
   mozzarella cheese

1. Preheat the oven to 240°C/220°C fan/475°F/ Gas mark 9, and line a large baking tray (sheet pan) with baking parchment.
2. Place the sweet potato circles onto the prepared baking tray.
3. Mix the tomato purée (paste) and mixed herbs in a small bowl.
4. Spread 1 teaspoon of the herby purée over each of the sweet potato slices, then sprinkle evenly with the grated mozzarella.
5. Place the melts into the oven to bake for about 15 minutes, or until the cheese is golden. Alternatively, air-fry at 200°C/400°F for 12 minutes.
6. Cut into finger-width slices and serve once cooled.

   Allergy swaps: For a dairy allergy, swap the cheese for a dairy-free Cheddar.

CARROTY PIZZA SOLDIERS

||||||||||||||||||||||||||||||||||||||||||||||||||||||||||||||||||||||||||||||||||||||||||||||

Few things are as comforting as these soldiers, brimming with the beloved flavours of pizza, but now elevated with the sweet addition of carrots. My little ones can't resist this recipe, and I'm sure yours will fall in love with it too. It's also a fantastic recipe for fussy eaters!

Prep + cook time: **8 mins**

MAKES 4 PORTIONS

4 tablespoons tomato purée (paste)

4 tablespoons unsalted butter, melted

2 teaspoons minced garlic

4 slices white bread

1 small carrot, grated

120g (4¼oz/1 cup) grated Cheddar cheese

1. Heat the grill to a medium heat.
2. In a small bowl, mix the tomato purée (paste), butter and minced garlic.
3. Spoon a quarter of the filling onto each slice of bread and spread it out evenly.
4. In a medium bowl, combine the grated carrot and cheese.
5. Sprinkle a quarter of the grated carrot and cheese evenly over each slice of bread.
6. Place the bread slices under the grill for 3–5 minutes, until golden brown and bubbling.
7. Slice into soldiers and serve once cooled.

Allergy swaps: For a dairy allergy, swap the butter for a dairy-free alternative, and swap the cheese for a dairy-free Cheddar. For a gluten intolerance, swap the bread for a gluten-free variety.

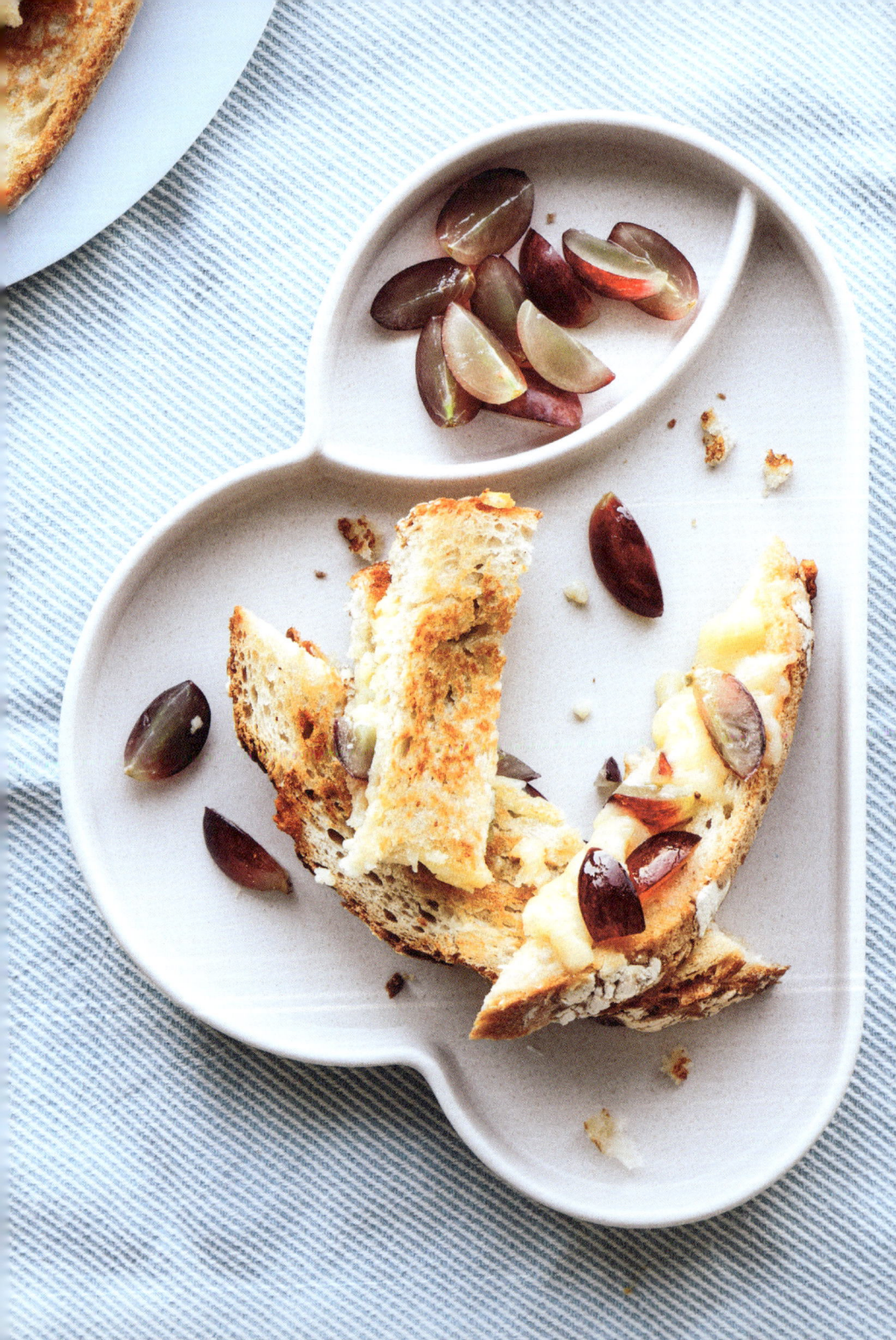

GRAPE AND CHEESE TOASTIE SOLDIERS

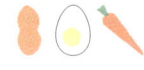

||||||||||||||||||||||||||||||||||||||||||||||||||||||||||||||||||||||||||||||||||||||||||||||||||||

Your baby will love indulging in the gooey comfort of this delicious toastie. It's an irresistible combination of sweet and savoury, and perfectly warming during the colder autumn and winter months.

Prep + cook time: **12 mins**

MAKES 2 PORTIONS

4 thick slices white bread
4 teaspoons unsalted
   butter, for spreading
120g (4oz/1 cup) grated
   Cheddar cheese
75g (2¾oz/½ cup) red
   seedless grapes,
   quartered lengthwise

1. Spread the slices of bread with a thin layer of unsalted butter.
2. In a small bowl, mix together the grated cheese and grapes, then spoon the mix evenly over 2 slices of the buttered bread.
3. Close the toasties by placing the remaining slices of bread on top, and carefully butter the outside of the toasties.
4. Heat a frying pan (skillet) over a low-medium heat and dry-fry the toasties for 2 minutes on each side, or until golden brown and oozy.
5. Slice into soldiers and serve once cooled.

Allergy swaps: For a gluten intolerance, swap the bread for a gluten-free variety. For a dairy allergy, swap the cheese for a dairy-free Cheddar, and swap the butter for a dairy-free alternative.

BEAN AND CHEESE TORTILLA

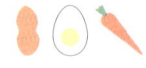

||||||||||||||||||||||||||||||||||||||||||||||||||||||||||||||||||||||||||||||||||||||||||||||||||||||||

This stuffed tortilla is the ultimate comfort lunch, packed with oozy cheese and baked beans in a rich, savoury sauce. Slice into long, finger-width strips so it's perfect for little hands to grip.

Prep + cook time: **17 mins**

MAKES 2 PORTIONS

1 x 200g (7oz) tin of low
   sugar and salt baked
   beans
1 small carrot, grated
2 large tortilla wraps
60g (2oz/½ cup) grated
   Cheddar cheese

1. Preheat the oven to 220°C/200°C fan/450°F/ Gas mark 8, and grease or line a baking tray (sheet pan) with baking parchment.
2. Add the baked beans to a shallow bowl and mash with the back of a fork. Once mashed, stir through the grated carrot.
3. Spoon half of the mix over one side of each tortilla, then top evenly with a sprinkling of grated cheese.
4. Fold the uncoated side of the wraps over the coated side to make a semi-circle.
5. Place the tortillas onto the prepared baking tray and bake in the oven for 10–12 minutes until they are golden and the cheese has melted inside. Alternatively, air-fry at 180°C/350°F for 8 minutes.
6. Slice into long, finger-width strips and serve once cooled.

   Allergy swaps: For a dairy allergy, swap the cheese for a dairy-free Cheddar. For a gluten intolerance, swap the tortilla wraps for a gluten-free variety or sweet potato wraps.

LEFTOVER VEGETABLE PINWHEELS

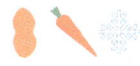

During the initial stages of baby-led weaning, you may find yourself with leftover vegetables, wondering how to put them to good use. Pastry pinwheels are a brilliant solution for repurposing them into a delectable savoury lunch.

Prep + cook time: **20 mins**

MAKES 10–12 PORTIONS

1 ready-rolled puff pastry sheet
3 tablespoons cream cheese
90g (3oz/1 cup) leftover cooked vegetables, roughly diced
60g (2oz/½ cup) grated Cheddar cheese
1 medium egg, beaten

1. Preheat the oven to 240°C/220°C fan/475°F/ Gas mark 9, and grease or line a baking tray (sheet pan) with baking parchment.
2. Unroll the puff pastry sheet and spread evenly with the cream cheese.
3. Sprinkle the diced vegetables and grated Cheddar over the cream cheese layer.
4. Re-roll the pastry sheet along the long edge to create a log shape.
5. Using a sharp knife, cut the log into 2.5cm (1in) pieces to create your pinwheels. If this makes too many, you can freeze some before cooking them.
6. Place your pinwheels onto the baking tray and brush with the beaten egg. Bake for 15 minutes, or until golden brown. Serve once cooled. Alternatively, air-fry at 200°C/400°F for 12 minutes.

Allergy swaps: For a dairy allergy, swap the cream cheese for a dairy-free soft cheese. For an egg allergy, swap the egg for 2 teaspoons vegetable oil. For a gluten intolerance, swap the puff pastry for a gluten-free variety.

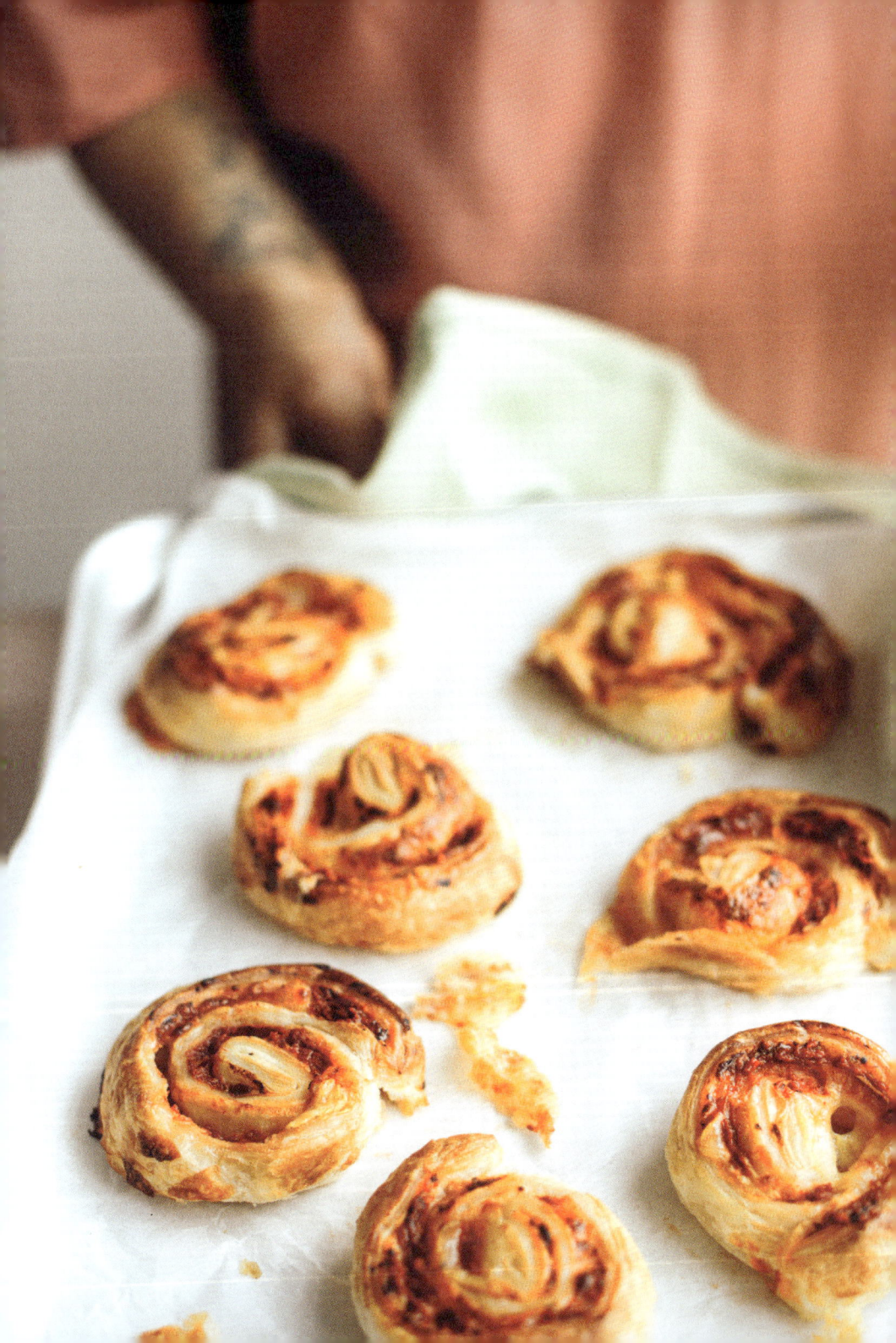

CHEESE AND COURGETTE PINWHEELS

|||||||||||||||||||||||||||||||||||||||||||||||||||||||||||||||||||||||||||||||||||||||||||||||||||

These mouthwatering pinwheels are a quick and hassle-free bite designed to delight your baby's tastebuds. An excellent choice for a speedy, wholesome lunch or a light dinner, they're bursting with flavour, family-friendly and they freeze exceptionally well, making them a convenient addition to your recipe arsenal.

Prep + cook time: **20 mins**

MAKES 10–12 PORTIONS

1 ready-rolled puff pastry sheet
3 tablespoons tomato purée (paste)
120g (4oz/1 cup) grated Cheddar cheese
1 small courgette (zucchini), grated and excess moisture squeezed out
2 teaspoons whole (full-fat) milk

1. Preheat the oven to 240°C/220°C fan/475°F/Gas mark 9, and grease or line a baking tray (sheet pan) with baking parchment.
2. Unroll the puff pastry sheet and spread evenly with the tomato purée (paste).
3. In a small bowl, mix the grated cheese and courgette (zucchini). Once combined, spoon this evenly over the tomato layer.
4. Re-roll the pastry sheet along the long edge to create a log shape.
5. Using a sharp knife, cut the log into 2.5cm (1in) pieces to create your pinwheels. If this makes too many, you can freeze some before cooking them.
6. Place your pinwheels onto the prepared baking tray and brush with the milk. Bake for 15 minutes, or until golden and slightly crisp. Serve once cooled. Alternatively, air-fry at 200°C/400°F for 12 minutes.

Allergy swaps: Swap the cheese for a dairy-free Cheddar, and swap the milk for soya, oat, coconut, breast or formula milk. For a gluten intolerance, swap the puff pastry for a gluten-free variety.

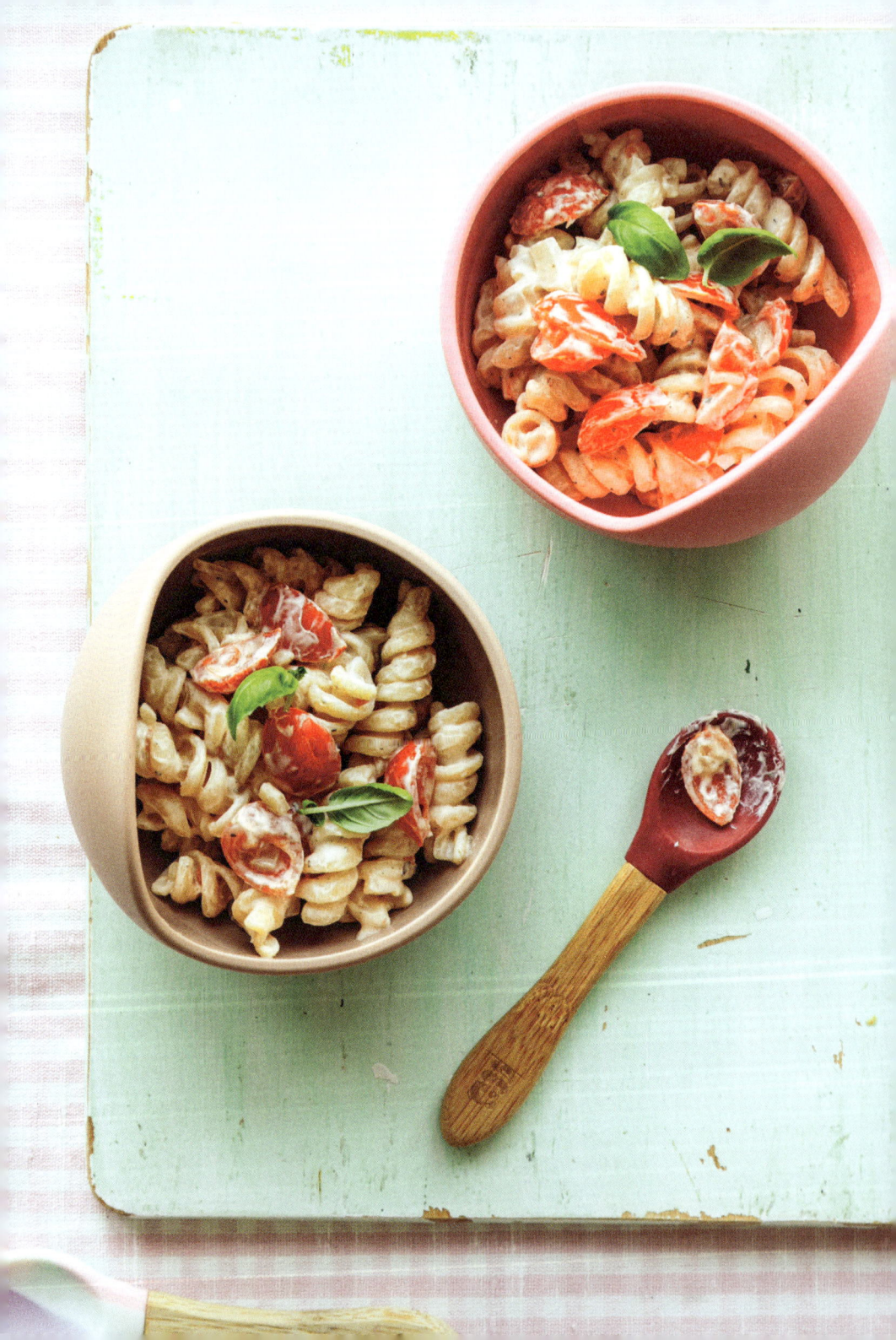

THE EASIEST CREAMIEST PASTA

|||||||||||||||||||||||||||||||||||||||||||||||||||||||||||||||||||||||||||||||||||||||||||||||||||||||||||||||||||

Enjoy the simplicity of this creamy pasta, crafted with just six ingredients. Cream cheese is a saviour for busy parents; versatile enough to enhance pasta, elevate toast or crackers, or serve as a dip for breadsticks. Its richness in both fat and calories positions it as a valuable addition to your baby's diet while also providing essential nutrients such as calcium, vitamin A and protein. For older children and adults, try frying some bacon lardons with the onion for extra yumminess.

Prep + cook time: **20 mins**

MAKES 4 PORTIONS

300g (10½oz/3 cups)
  fusilli pasta
1 teaspoon vegetable oil
1 onion, very finely diced
200g (7oz/1⅓ cup) garlic
  and herb cream cheese
100ml (3½fl oz/
  scant ½ cup) whole
  (full-fat) milk
250g (9oz/1⅔ cups
  cherry tomatoes,
  sliced into quarters

1. Set a large saucepan of water on the hob over a high heat. Once the water is boiling, carefully add the pasta and reduce the heat to a gentle simmer. Cook the pasta according to the packet instructions, for around 12 minutes.
2. While the pasta cooks, heat the oil in a small frying pan (skillet) over a low-medium heat and fry the onions until soft.
3. Drain the pasta and return it to the empty saucepan. Stir through the fried onion, cream cheese, milk and cherry tomatoes and warm over a low heat for 3 minutes until the ingredients are well combined. Serve and enjoy once cooled.

Allergy swaps: For a dairy allergy, swap the cream cheese for a dairy-free soft cheese mixed with 2 teaspoons mixed herbs and 1 teaspoon minced garlic, and swap the milk for soya, oat, coconut, breast or formula milk. For a gluten intolerance, swap the pasta for gluten-free.

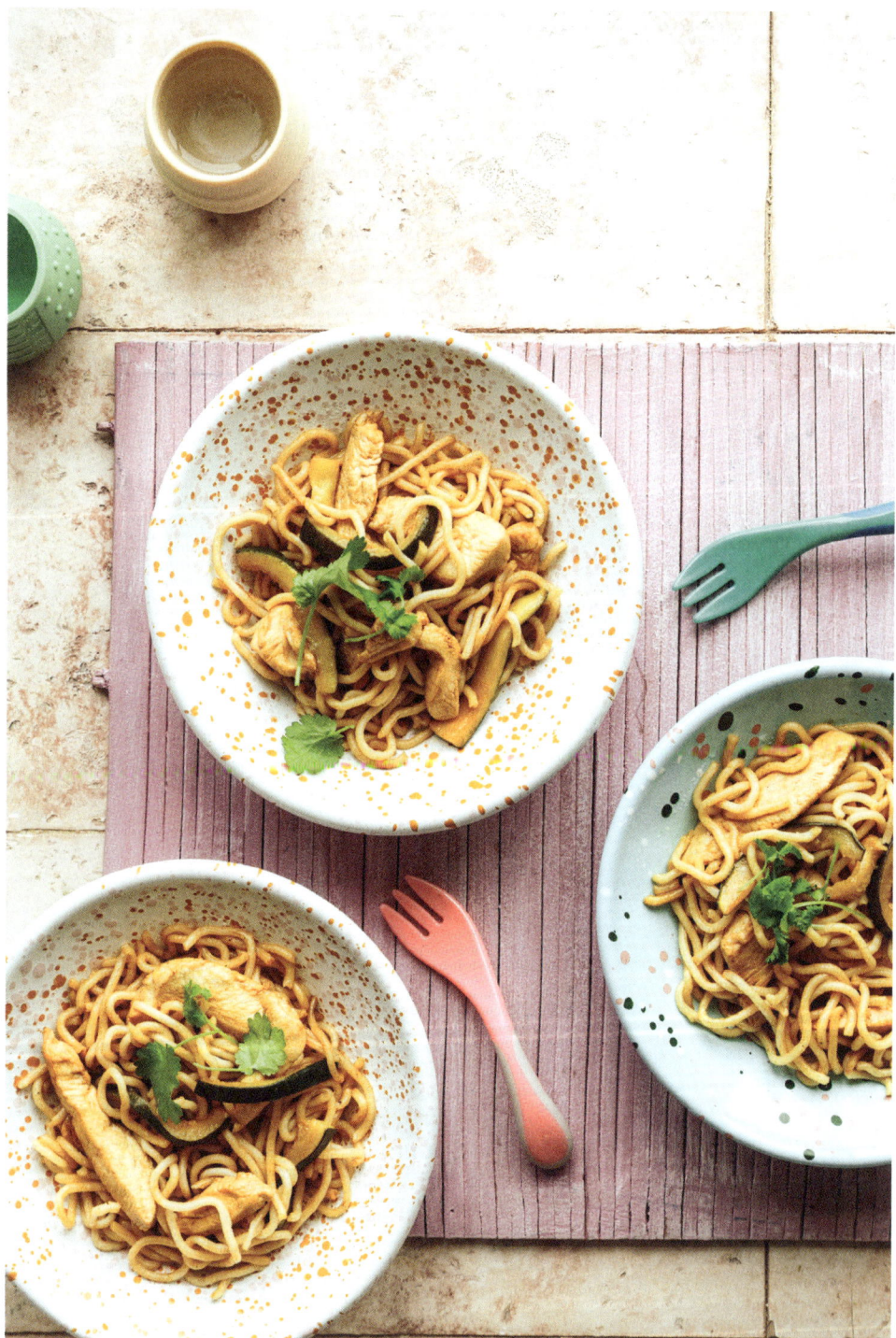

QUICK CHICKEN STIR FRY

This stir fry is the perfect tasty and nutritious family meal for busy days when you need something quick and satisfying.

Prep + cook time: **18 mins**

MAKES 4 PORTIONS

1 teaspoon vegetable oil
250g (9oz) chicken breasts, thinly sliced
1 medium courgette (zucchini), sliced into finger-width batons
1 teaspoon minced garlic
2 tablespoons reduced-salt soy sauce
60ml (2fl oz/¼ cup) orange juice
2 x 150g (5oz) packs of 'straight to wok' noodles

1. Heat the vegetable oil in a wok or large frying pan (skillet) over a medium heat.
2. Add the sliced chicken and fry for 5 minutes until fully cooked through.
3. Add the courgette (zucchini) and fry for another 3 minutes.
4. Finally, add the garlic, soy sauce, orange juice and noodles and fry for a final 5 minutes. Serve once cooled.

Allergy swaps: For a gluten intolerance, swap the noodles for a rice noodle variety, ensuring it is 100% gluten free.

BROCCOLI LEMON CHICKEN

A zesty one-pan wonder! Like all of my recipes, it's ideal for every age group, but it's especially good for baby-led weaning because it includes long, juicy chicken strips and tender broccoli florets, which are easy for babies to pick up and hold.

Prep + cook time: **20 mins**

MAKES 2 PORTIONS

1 tablespoon vegetable oil
300g (10½oz) chicken
   breast, thinly sliced
2 teaspoons minced garlic
300g (10½oz/3 cups)
   fresh or frozen broccoli
250ml (8½fl oz/1 cup)
   low-salt chicken stock
   (broth)
2 tablespoons cornflour
   (cornstarch)
1 tablespoon maple syrup
   (optional)
Potato wedges or rice,
   to serve

1. Heat the oil in a large frying pan (skillet) or wok over a medium heat, then add the chicken and fry for 3 minutes.
2. Add the minced garlic and broccoli and fry for a further 2 minutes.
3. Mix the stock (broth), cornflour (cornstarch) and maple syrup (if using) in a jug (pitcher), then pour into the pan and simmer for 10 minutes until the sauce has thickened and the chicken is cooked through.
4. Leave to cool slightly, and enjoy with some potato wedges or rice.

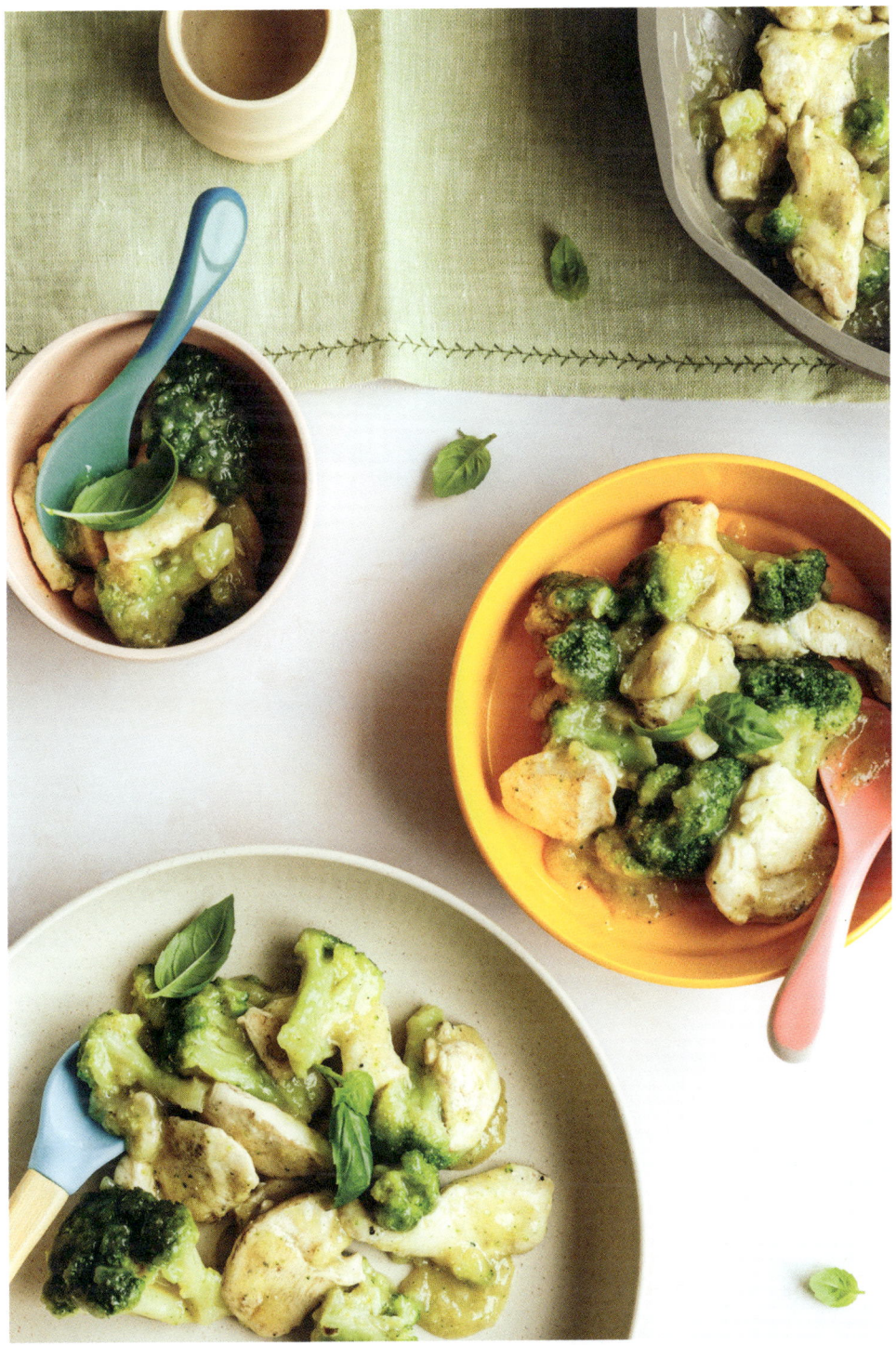

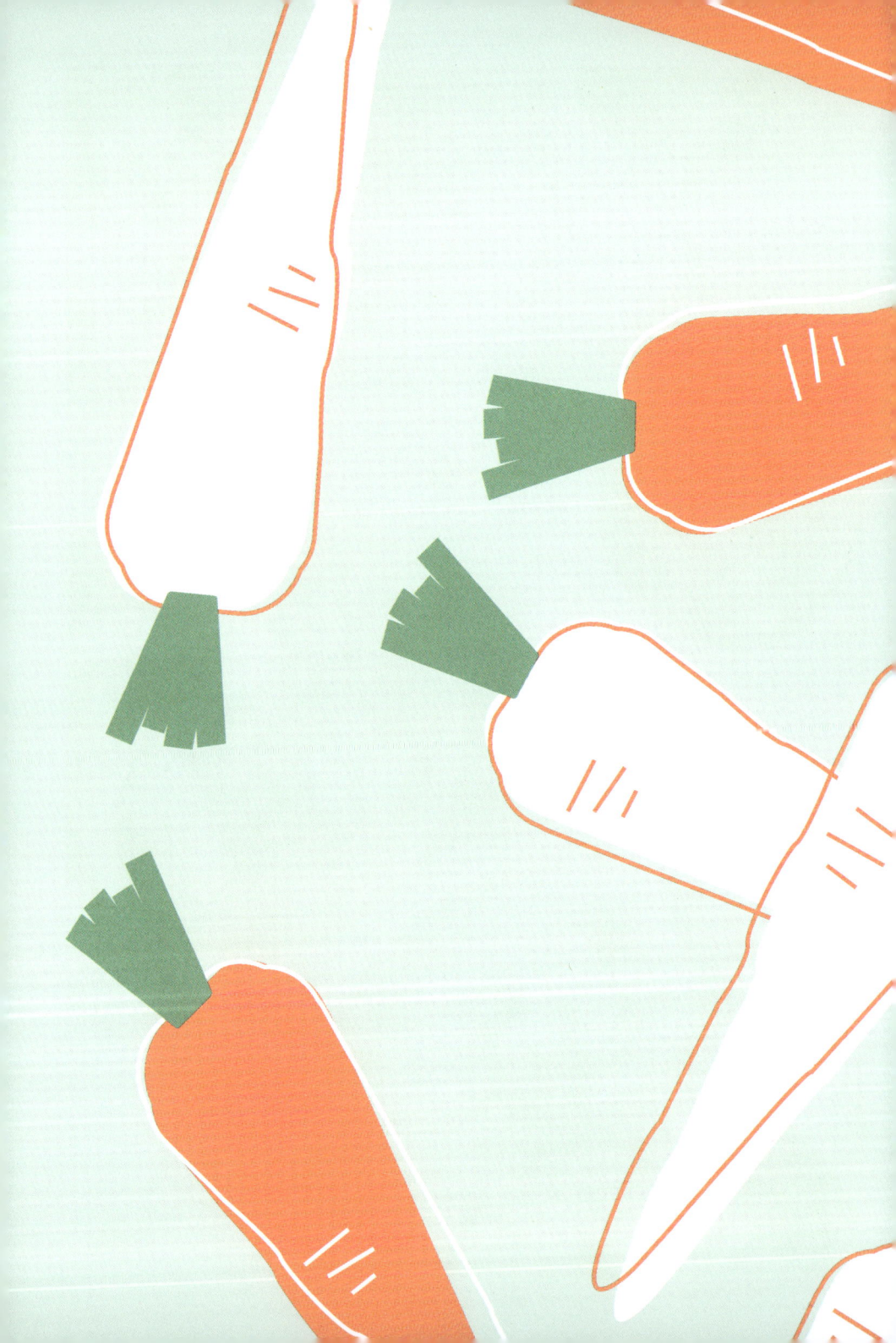

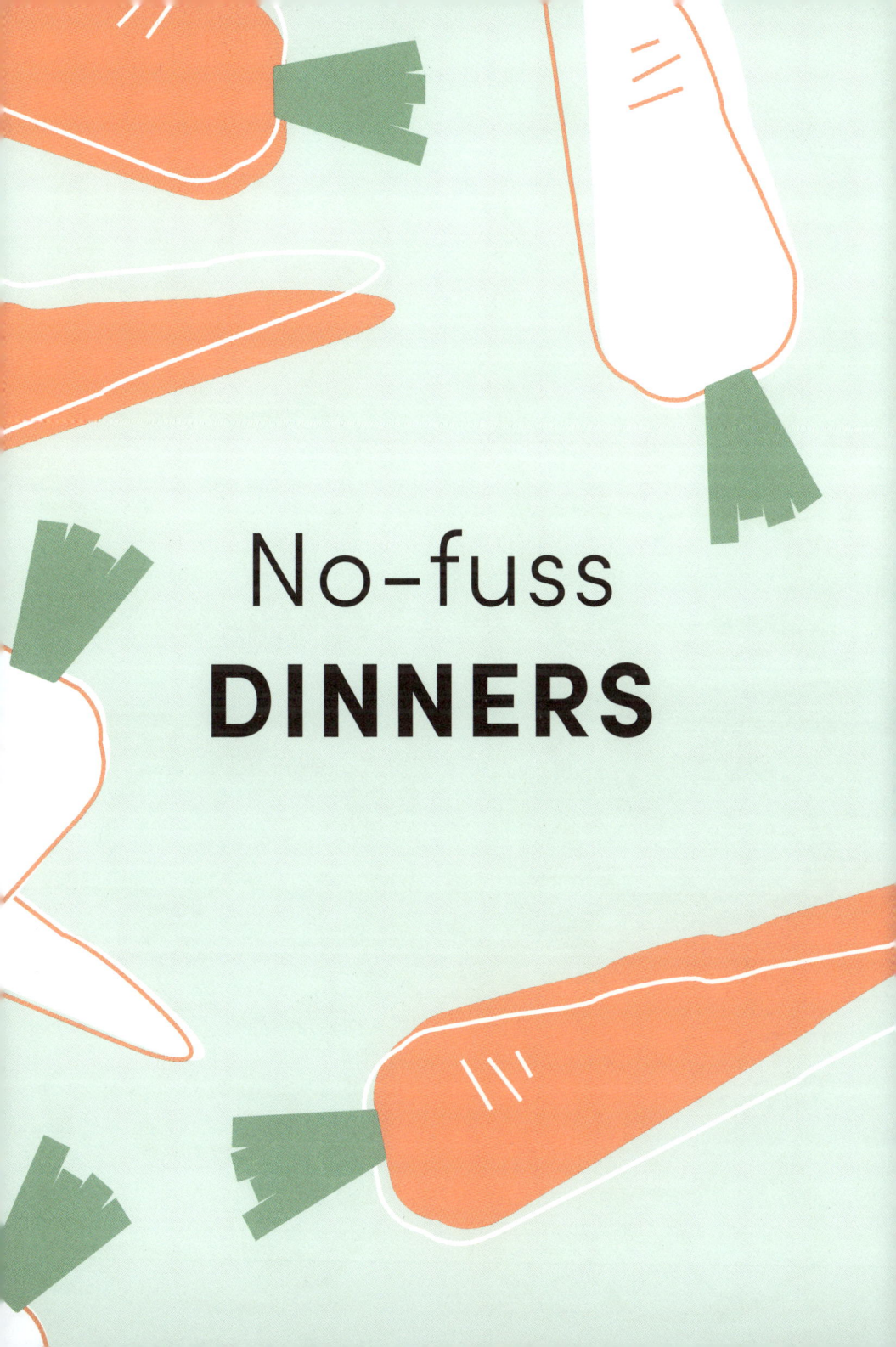

No-fuss
DINNERS

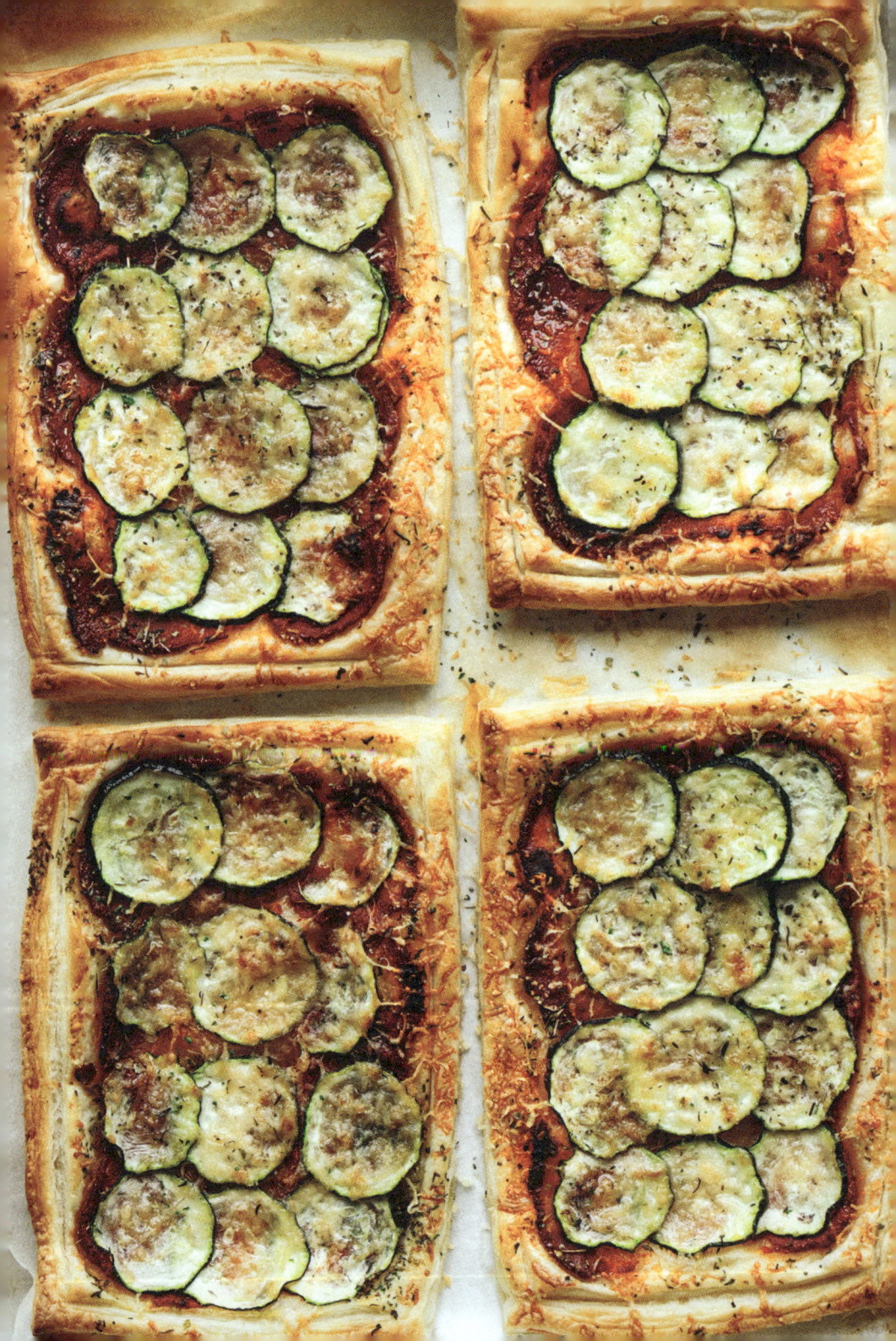

COURGETTE TARTS

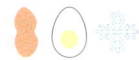

||||||||||||||||||||||||||||||||||||||||||||||||||||||||||||||||||||||||||||||||||||||||||||||

Whipping up this tasty courgette (zucchini) tart is a breeze. It's a flaky, veggie-packed delight that's perfect for lazy lunches or quick dinners, so dig in!

Prep + cook time: **20 mins**

MAKES 4 PORTIONS

1 ready-rolled puff
    pastry sheet
4 teaspoons tomato
    purée (paste)
1 teaspoon mixed herbs
½ small courgette
    (zucchini), very finely
    sliced
2 tablespoons grated
    Parmesan cheese

1. Preheat the oven to 240°C/220°C fan/475°F/
   Gas mark 9, and place the pastry sheet, complete
   with baking parchment, onto a large baking tray
   (sheet pan).
2. Cut the pastry sheet into quarters to create
   4 rectangles, then score a 5mm (¼in) border around
   each one.
3. Spread 1 teaspoon of tomato purée (paste) over
   each tart and sprinkle each with a ¼ teaspoon
   of mixed herbs.
4. Add a layer of sliced courgette (zucchini) over the
   top of each tart.
5. Finally, sprinkle each tart evenly with the Parmesan
   cheese.
6. Place the tarts into the oven to bake for
   12–15 minutes until golden. Serve once cooled.
   Alternatively, air-fry at 200°C/400°F for 12 minutes.

   Allergy swaps: For a dairy allergy, swap the
   Parmesan for a dairy-free Parmesan. For a gluten
   intolerance, swap the puff pastry for a gluten-free
   variety.

NO-EFFORT NAAN PIZZA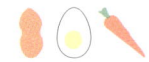

This pizza is the ultimate lazy-day dinner hack that tastes anything but lazy. Grab some naan bread, pile on your favourite toppings and in no time at all you'll have a mouthwatering pizza ready for your family to devour.

Prep + cook time: **15 mins**

MAKES 2 PORTIONS

2 naan breads
2 tablespoons tomato
  purée (paste)
120g (4¼oz/1 cup) grated
  mozzarella cheese
6 cherry tomatoes, sliced
  into quarters

1. Preheat the oven to 220°C/200°C fan/450°F/Gas mark 8, and line a large baking tray (sheet pan) with baking parchment.
2. Place the naan breads onto the prepared baking tray, then spread each naan with 1 tablespoon of tomato purée (paste) and top with the mozzarella and quartered cherry tomatoes.
3. Place the naan breads into the oven and cook for 8–10 minutes until the mozzarella is golden and oozy. Slice and serve once cooled. Alternatively, air-fry at 180°C/350°F for 8 minutes.

Allergy swaps: For a dairy-free alternative, swap the cheese for a dairy-free variety. For a gluten intolerance, swap the naan breads for gluten-free pizza bases or bread.

NOTE

You can easily adapt this recipe with your family's favourite toppings. Alternative options could include diced mushrooms, diced (bell) peppers, sliced chicken or pineapple.

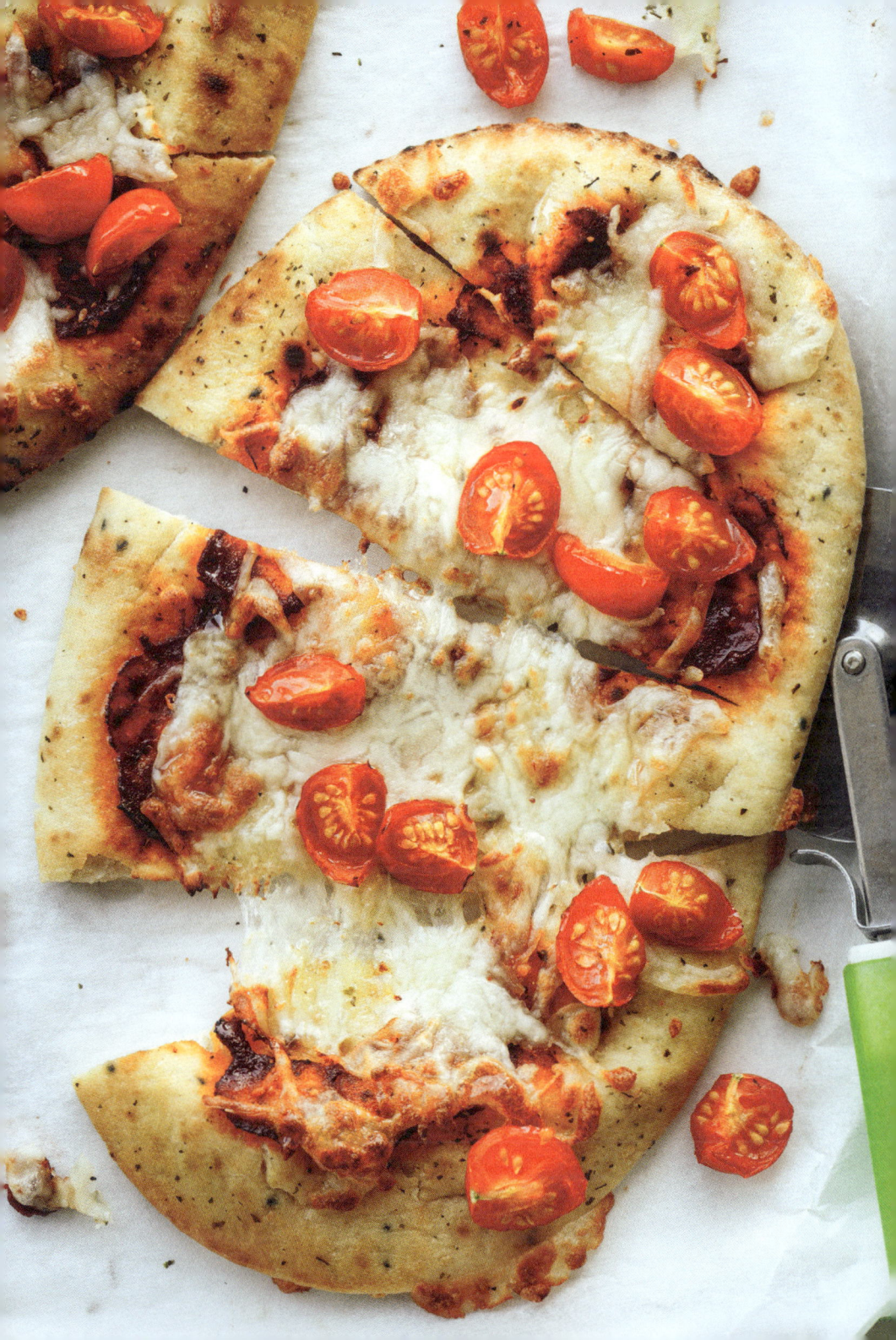

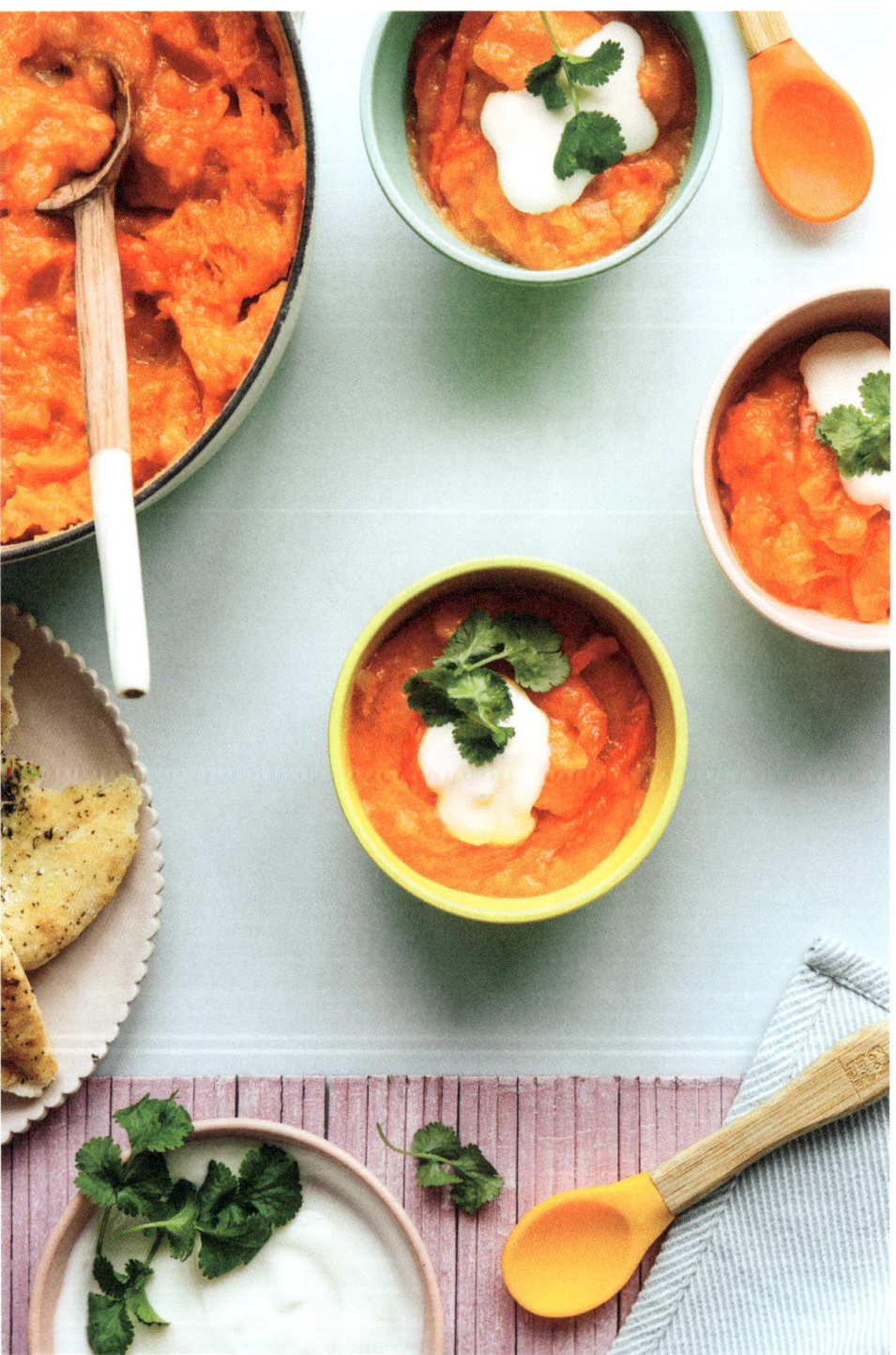

BUTTERNUT SQUASH THAI CURRY

||||||||||||||||||||||||||||||||||||||||||||||||||||||||||||||||||||||||||||||||||||||||||||||||||||||||||||||||

If your family loves curry and has a sweet tooth, this will be a match made in heaven for you. The natural sweetness of butternut squash complements the bold and aromatic red curry spices, resulting in a comforting and satisfying curry.

Prep + cook time: **20 mins**

MAKES 4 PORTIONS

1 teaspoon vegetable oil
1 onion, finely diced
1 red (bell) pepper, deseeded and thinly sliced
250g (9oz/2 cups) frozen butternut squash chunks
1 x 400g (14oz) tin of coconut milk
2 tablespoons Thai red curry paste (see Note, page 154)
Full-fat natural yoghurt, to serve
Chunky bread or naan, for dipping

1. Heat the oil in a large saucepan over a medium-high heat and fry the onion and red pepper for 2 minutes.
2. Add the butternut squash, coconut milk and Thai red curry paste and simmer for 13 minutes, or until the butternut squash is soft and cooked through.
3. Once cooked, test the spiciness of the dish and stir as much yoghurt as needed into each portion as you serve.
4. Serve once cooled with some slices of chunky bread or naan for dipping.

Allergy swaps: For a dairy allergy, swap the yoghurt for a soya, coconut or oat alternative. For a gluten intolerance, swap the bread for a gluten-free variety or serve with rice instead.

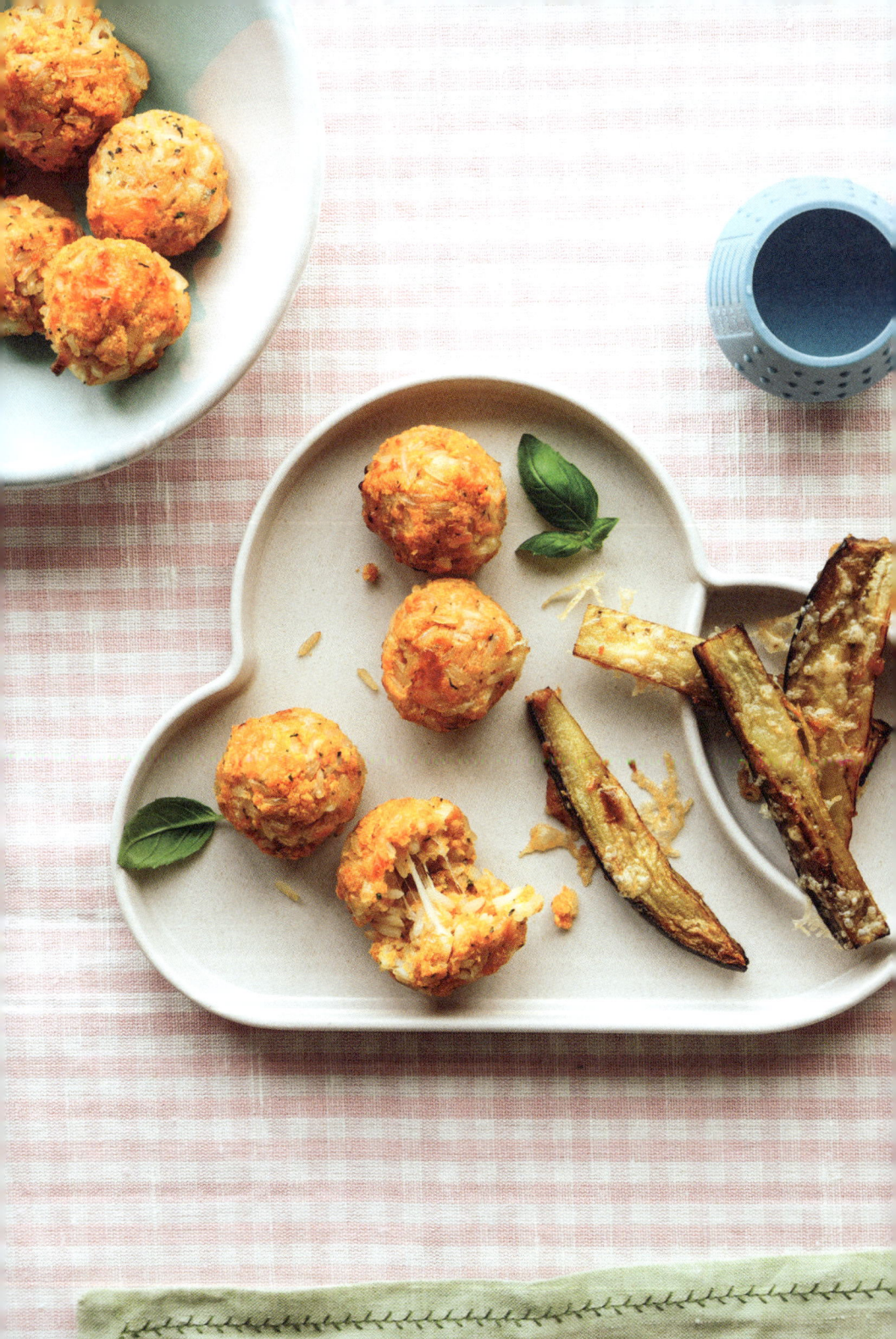

RICE BALLS WITH CRISPY AUBERGINE CHIPS

These mini bites are a flavour-packed adventure, perfect for little hands. I've paired the delicious rice balls with crispy aubergine (eggplant) chips for extra crunch

Prep + cook time: **20 mins**

MAKES 3 PORTIONS

1 x 250g (9oz) packet
of long-grain
microwave rice
100g (3½oz/1 cup)
golden breadcrumbs
120g (4¼oz/1 cup) grated
mozzarella cheese
2 medium eggs
1½ teaspoons dried
mixed herbs
1 aubergine (eggplant),
sliced into finger-sized
batons
1 tablespoon olive oil
2 tablespoons grated
Parmesan cheese

1. Preheat the oven to 240°C/220°C fan/475°F/Gas mark 9, and line 2 large baking trays (sheet pans) with baking parchment.
2. Place the rice, breadcrumbs, cheese, eggs and mixed herbs in a large mixing bowl and stir well to combine.
3. Take heaped tablespoons of the rice mix and roll them into tightly packed golf-ball-sized balls, placing them on one of the prepared baking trays as you go.
4. In another bowl, add the aubergine (eggplant) chips, olive oil and Parmesan and toss together until the aubergine chips are evenly coated.
5. Transfer the aubergine onto the remaining baking tray and spread out evenly.
6. Place both the rice balls and aubergine chips into the oven and cook for 15 minutes, or until golden. Serve once cooled. Alternatively, air-fry at 200°C/400°F for 12 minutes.

Allergy swaps: Swap the cheeses for a dairy-free Parmesan and mozzarella. For a gluten intolerance, swap the breadcrumbs for gluten-free breadcrumbs, crushed gluten-free cornflakes or puffed rice cereal.

EASY-PEASY ROASTED PEPPER AND SPINACH PASTA

sauce only

This pasta dish calls for minimal preparation, making it a go-to option for a stress-free weeknight dinner. It's also a fantastic way to get iron-rich spinach into your baby's diet!

Prep + cook time: **15 mins**

MAKES 4 PORTIONS

300g (10½oz/3 cups) dried pasta of your choice
200g (7oz) jar of roasted red peppers (including the oil)
3 handfuls of baby spinach
3 teaspoons minced garlic
125ml (4¼fl oz/½ cup) double (heavy) cream
1 teaspoon dried mixed herbs
Pinch of smoked paprika

1. Set a large saucepan of water on the hob over a high heat. Once the water is boiling, add the pasta and reduce the heat to a gentle simmer. Cook the pasta according to the packet instructions, for around 12 minutes.
2. While the pasta cooks, add the remaining ingredients to a blender or food processor and blend to form a smooth sauce.
3. Drain the pasta, return it to the pan and stir through the creamy pepper sauce. Warm through over a low heat for 1–2 minutes, then serve once cooled.

Allergy swaps: For a gluten intolerance, swap the pasta for a gluten-free variety. For a dairy allergy, swap the cream for a dairy-free alternative.

COCONUT CHICKEN NOODLES

||||||||||||||||||||||||||||||||||||||||||||||||||||||||||||||||||||||||||||||||||||||||||||||||

Get ready for a tastebud adventure with my yummy chicken noodles. A magical blend of exotic flavours in a fun, slurp-worthy sauce!

Prep + cook time: **20 mins**

MAKES 4 PORTIONS

1 teaspoon vegetable oil
1 onion, *thinly sliced*
1 red (bell) pepper, *deseeded and thinly sliced*
300g (10½oz) chicken breasts, *thinly sliced*
1 teaspoon smoked paprika
2 teaspoons minced garlic
½ teaspoon minced ginger
2 tablespoons tomato purée (paste)
250g (9oz/1 cup) coconut cream
125g (4½oz) egg noodle nests

1. Heat the oil in a large frying pan (skillet) over a medium-high heat, then add the onions and peppers and fry for 5 minutes until softened.
2. Add the sliced chicken, paprika, garlic and ginger and fry for a further 5 minutes, or until the chicken is fully cooked through.
3. Add the tomato purée (paste), coconut cream and noodles, and simmer for a further 5 minutes, stirring until the noodles are soft and well coated in the sauce. Break the noodles down slightly with your spoon to help them along. Serve once cooled.

Allergy swaps: For a gluten intolerance, swap the noodles for a gluten-free variety or use rice instead. For an egg allergy, swap for rice noodles.

ONE-PAN COD CURRY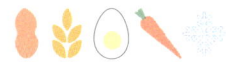

Discover the delight of a 20-minute fish curry – the ultimate solution for hectic days when you crave a nourishing meal for your little one without a lot of hassle or washing up. This is a luscious, velvety and heartwarming dish, perfect for a family dinner. For grown-ups, a small pinch of salt really elevates the dish.

Prep + cook time: **20 mins**

MAKES 4 PORTIONS

1 teaspoon vegetable oil
3 yellow (bell) peppers, deseeded and very thinly sliced
2 teaspoons minced garlic
2 x 400ml (14oz) tins of coconut milk
1 tablespoon Thai red curry paste (see Note)
1 tablespoon tomato purée (paste)
1 tablespoon maple syrup (optional)
Pinch of ground black pepper
4 x 125g cod fillets sliced
Full-fat natural yoghurt, to serve

1. Heat the oil in a large saucepan over a high heat. Add the peppers and garlic and fry for 5 minutes until softened.
2. Add the remaining ingredients, except the yoghurt, to the saucepan and stir gently to combine. Lower the heat to medium and let the dish simmer gently for 10 minutes, or until the cod is cooked through and starting to flake.
3. Once cooked, test the spiciness of the dish and stir as much yoghurt as needed into each portion as you serve (see Note).

Allergy swaps: For a dairy allergy, swap the yoghurt for a soya, coconut or oat alternative.

NOTE

The spice and salt levels of Thai red curry pastes can vary between brands. You may not need to add yoghurt, or you may need to add several tablespoons. Some babies love spice – experiment, and test your baby's reaction.

This curry is great served with rice – for babies, I recommend stirring the rice into the curry to make it thicker, so it's easier to grip.

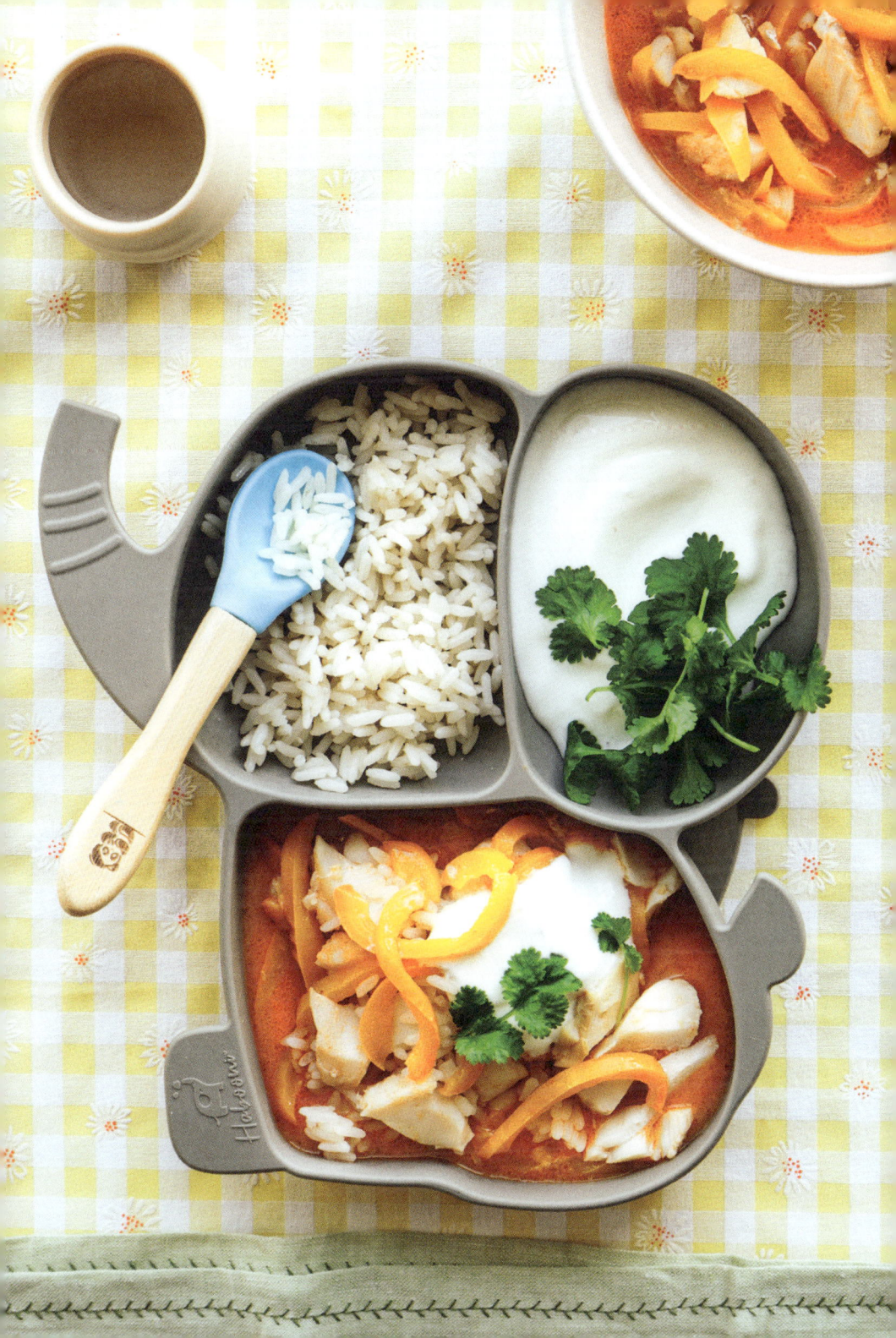

EASY BURGER WRAPS

Imagine your favourite burger wrapped snugly in a warm, comforting tortilla . . . Your family will fall head over heels for this mouthwatering recipe. Plus, as your little one grows, it's a fantastic opportunity for them to get creative with additional fillings – gherkins ahoy!

Prep + cook time: **20 mins**

MAKES 4 PORTIONS

4 large tortilla wraps
500g (1lb 2oz/generous
    2 cups) minced (ground)
    beef (see Tip)
2 salad tomatoes,
    finely diced
120g (4¼oz/1 cup)
    mature Cheddar cheese
3 teaspoons dried
    mixed herbs
2 teaspoons minced garlic

Allergy swaps: For a dairy allergy, swap the cheese for a dairy-free Cheddar. For a gluten intolerance, swap the tortilla wraps for a gluten-free variety or sweet potato wraps.

1. Preheat the oven to 220°C/200°C fan/450°F/Gas mark 8, and line 2 large baking trays (sheet pans) with baking parchment.
2. Place 2 tortillas on each baking tray.
3. Add all the remaining ingredients to a mixing bowl and stir well to combine.
4. Divide the mince mixture evenly into 4, and roll each one into a burger ball, then place 1 ball in the centre of each tortilla.
5. Press the burger balls down with the palm of your hand, and use your hands to spread them out so they evenly coat the full surface of each tortilla.
6. Bake the tortillas in the oven for 15 minutes, or until the mince has browned and is completely cooked through. Alternatively, air-fry at 180°C/350°F for 12 minutes.
7. Carefully fold in half while still hot (using a fish slice and dish towel will help to protect your hands), then slice into finger-width strips and serve once cooled.

NOTE

Grown-ups and older children can add shredded lettuce, sliced red onions, gherkins and burger sauce. I recommend using a mince with 10% fat or less so that the wraps are not too greasy.

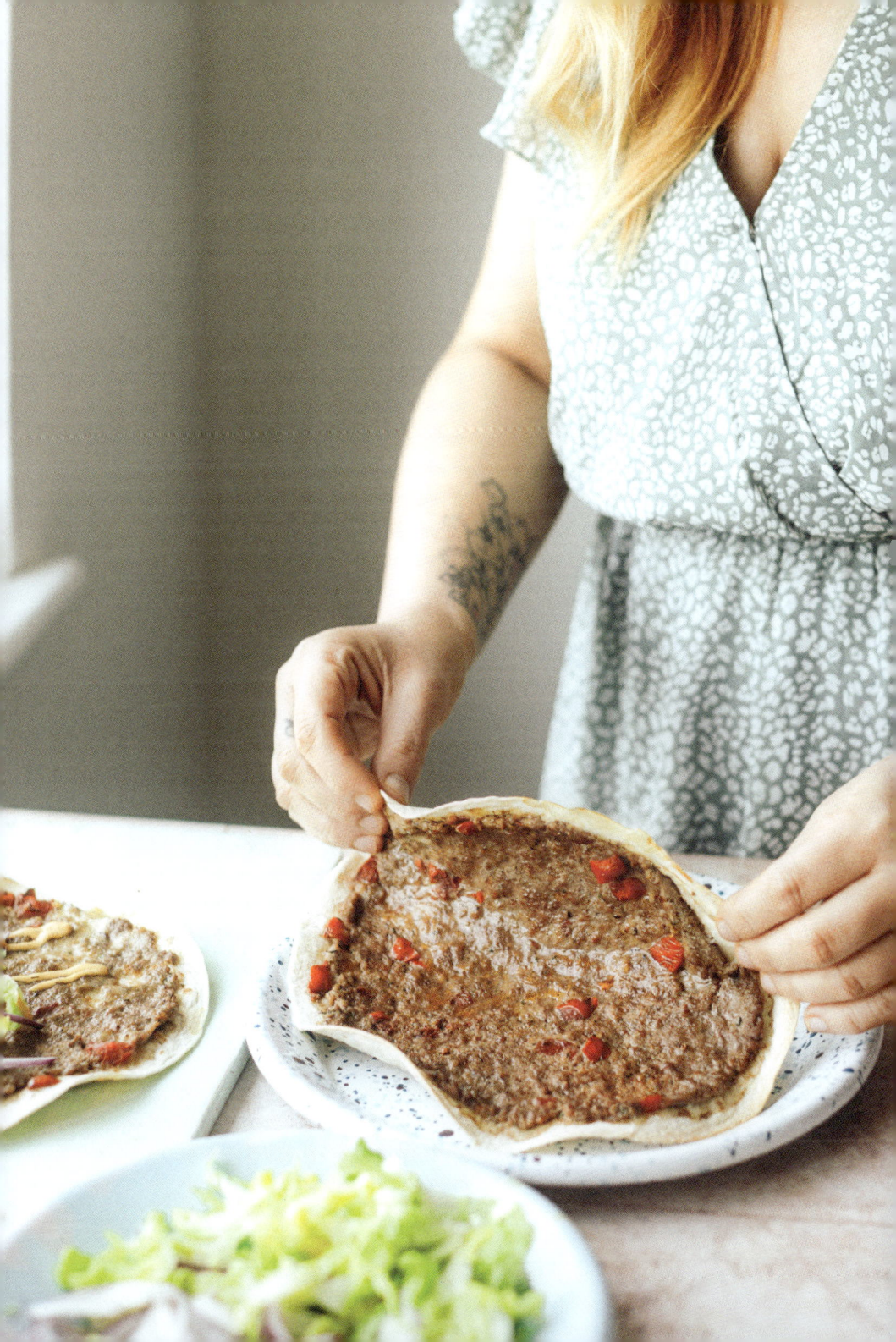

SUCCULENT CHICKEN BURGERS

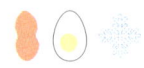

|||||||||||||||||||||||||||||||||||||||||||||||||||||||||||||||||||||||||||||||||||||||||||

A succulent chicken patty tucked inside a fluffy bun – but don't worry, this isn't a chef-only zone. This is a meal that's easy-peasy to whip up, even for kitchen rookies. So grab those burger buns and let's get cooking!

Prep + cook time: **17 mins**

MAKES 6 PORTIONS

500g (1lb 2oz/generous
    2 cups) minced (ground)
    chicken
60ml (2fl oz/¼ cup) Greek
    yoghurt
180g (6½oz/2 cups) oats
2 teaspoons minced garlic
3 teaspoons dried
    mixed herbs
½ teaspoon English
    mustard
1 tablespoon vegetable oil
4 burger buns

1. Place the chicken mince, Greek yoghurt, oats, garlic, herbs and mustard in a large mixing bowl and stir well to combine.
2. Divide the mix evenly into 6, then shape into burger patties, about 1cm (½in) thick.
3. Heat the oil in a frying pan (skillet) over a medium-high heat, and once hot, add the chicken burgers and fry for 5–6 minutes on each side until golden brown and fully cooked through.
4. Allow to cool, then serve in burger buns, cut into finger-width slices.

Allergy swaps: For a dairy allergy, swap the yoghurt for a soya, coconut or oat alternative. For a gluten intolerance, swap the oats and burger buns for gluten-free varieties.

NOTE

Grown-ups and older children can add fillings such as shredded lettuce, sliced red onions, sliced tomatoes, gherkins and garlic mayo sauce.

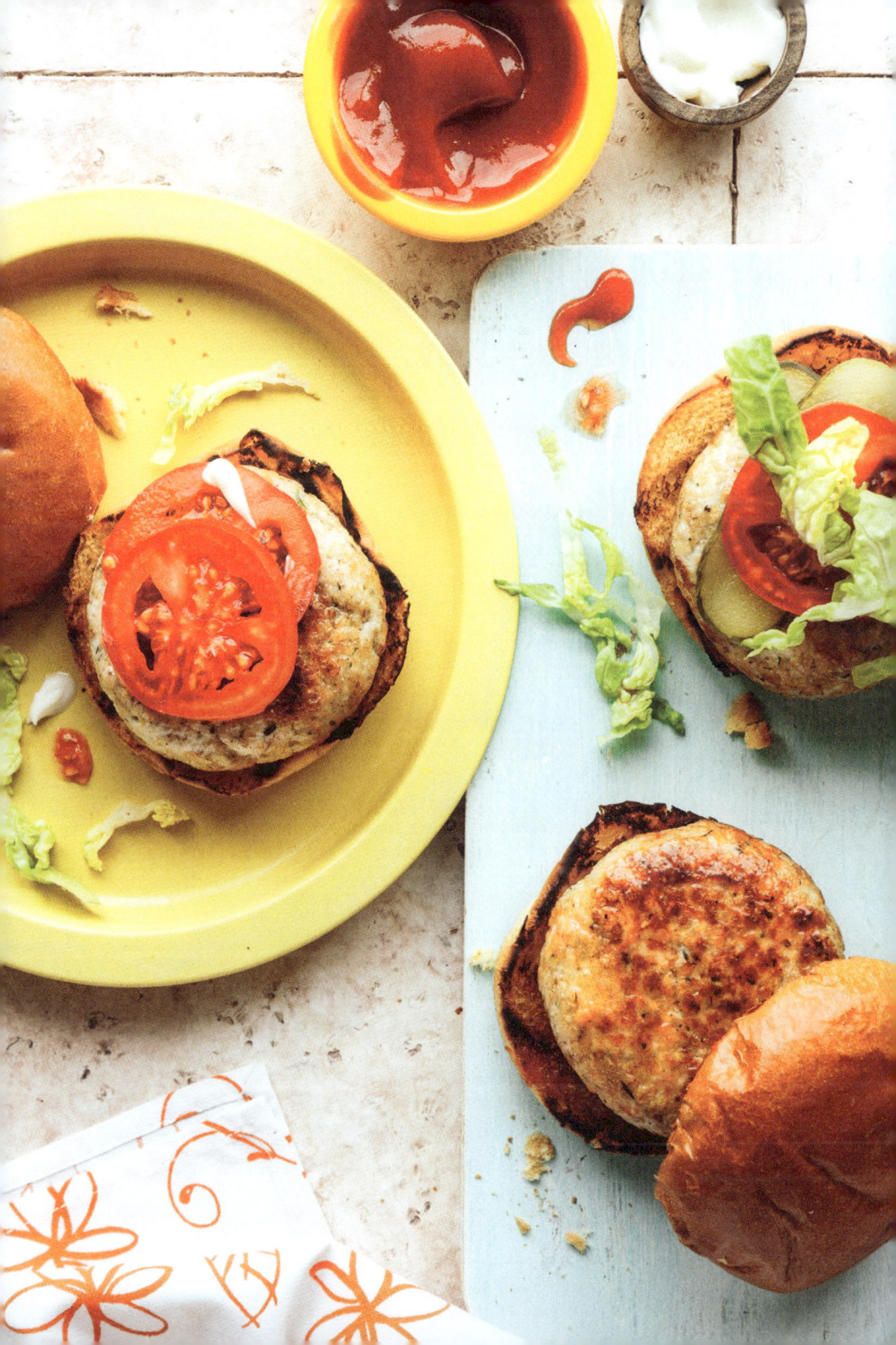

VEGETABLE-FILLED BEEF BURGERS

||||||||||||||||||||||||||||||||||||||||||||||||||||||||||||||||||||||||||||||||||||||||||

These juicy burgers are packed with vegetable goodness and a generous helping of sharp Cheddar cheese. They are perfect for the whole family to enjoy, and, when cut into strips, are ideal for little ones to grip and tuck in to!

Prep + cook time: **15 mins**

MAKES 10 PORTIONS

1 onion, roughly chopped
2 carrots, roughly chopped
100g (3½oz/1 cup)
    mushrooms, roughly
    chopped
90g (3oz/1 cup) grated
    Cheddar cheese
500g (1lb 2oz/generous
    2 cups) minced
    (ground) beef
60g (2oz/½ cup) dried
    breadcrumbs
1 medium egg, beaten
10 burger buns

1. Preheat a grill (broiler) to a high heat.
2. Place the onion, carrots and mushrooms in a food processor and blitz until the vegetables have broken down into small pieces, the size of coarse salt.
3. Spoon the chopped vegetables into a large mixing bowl and stir through the grated cheese, minced (ground) beef, breadcrumbs and egg.
4. Divide the mixture evenly into 10, and shape each one into a burger patty, about 5mm (¼in) thick.
5. Place the burgers on the grill tray and cook under the grill for about 10 minutes, very carefully flipping them after 5 minutes with the aid of a fish slice. Once cooked, the burgers will be golden brown, bubbling and fully cooked through, with no pink remaining.
6. Once cooled, serve in a fluffy burger bun, cut into finger-width slices.

Allergy swaps: Swap the cheese for a dairy-free Cheddar. Swap the egg for 1 tablespoon ground flaxseed stirred into 3 tablespoons water. Swap the breadcrumbs for gluten-free breadcrumbs, crushed gluten-free cornflakes or puffed rice cereal. Swap the burger buns for a gluten-free variety.

LAZY LASAGNE

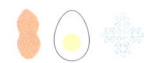

Lasagne holds a special place in my family's heart as the ultimate comfort food. However, as my family has grown and time has become more limited, I've yearned for a simpler version that offers the same comfort without the extensive prep time. So let me introduce you to my latest creation – a clever and time-saving twist on the ultimate cosy classic.

Prep + cook time: **20 mins**

MAKES 4 PORTIONS

1 teaspoon vegetable oil
1 onion, finely diced
2 carrots, very finely diced
500g (1lb 2oz/generous
   2 cups) minced
   (ground) beef
500ml (17fl oz/2 cups)
   low-salt beef stock
1 x 400g (14oz) tin of
   chopped tomatoes
1 teaspoon minced garlic
1 teaspoon dried
   mixed herbs
300g (10½oz) lasagne
   sheets, broken into
   shards
4 tablespoons cream
   cheese
3 tablespoons grated
   Parmesan cheese

1. Heat the oil in a large saucepan over a medium heat. Once hot, add the onion, carrots and mince and fry for 5 minutes, or until the mince has browned and the vegetables are soft.

2. Add the beef stock, chopped tomatoes, garlic, mixed herbs and broken lasagne sheets and simmer for 10 minutes, stirring occasionally.

3. Turn off the heat and stir through the cream cheese and Parmesan to create a rich, creamy sauce. Serve once cooled.

Allergy swaps: For a dairy allergy, swap the cream cheese and Parmesan for a dairy-free soft cheese and a dairy-free Parmesan. For a gluten intolerance, swap the pasta sheets for a gluten-free variety. For an egg allergy, double check the lasagne sheets do not contain egg.

GREEK LAMB SAUSAGES

Turn your baby's dinner into a Mediterranean feast with Greek lamb sausages – delicious paired with a dollop of thick, creamy Greek yoghurt, rice and salad.

Prep + cook time: **20 mins**

MAKES 4 PORTIONS

500g (1lb 2oz/generous 2 cups) minced (ground) lamb
1 red onion, very finely diced
2 teaspoons minced garlic
1 teaspoon ground cinnamon
1 teaspoon dried oregano
1 medium egg
50g (1¾oz/½ cup) dried breadcrumbs
Greek yoghurt, to serve (optional)

1. Preheat the oven to 250°C/230°C fan/480°F/Gas mark 9, and line a large baking tray (sheet pan) with baking parchment.
2. Add all the ingredients, except the yoghurt, to a large mixing bowl and stir well to combine.
3. Take 2 heaped tablespoons of the mix and roll it into a sausage shape, placing it onto the prepared baking tray. Repeat with the remaining mixture.
4. Place the sausages into the oven and cook for 15 minutes, or until browned and fully cooked through.
5. Serve once cooled with some creamy Greek yoghurt (if using) for dipping.

Allergy swaps: For a dairy allergy, swap the Greek yoghurt for a soya, coconut or oat alternative. For a gluten intolerance, swap the breadcrumbs for gluten-free breadcrumbs or crushed gluten-free cornflakes or puffed rice cereal. For an egg allergy, swap the egg for 1 tablespoon ground flaxseed stirred into 3 tablespoons water.

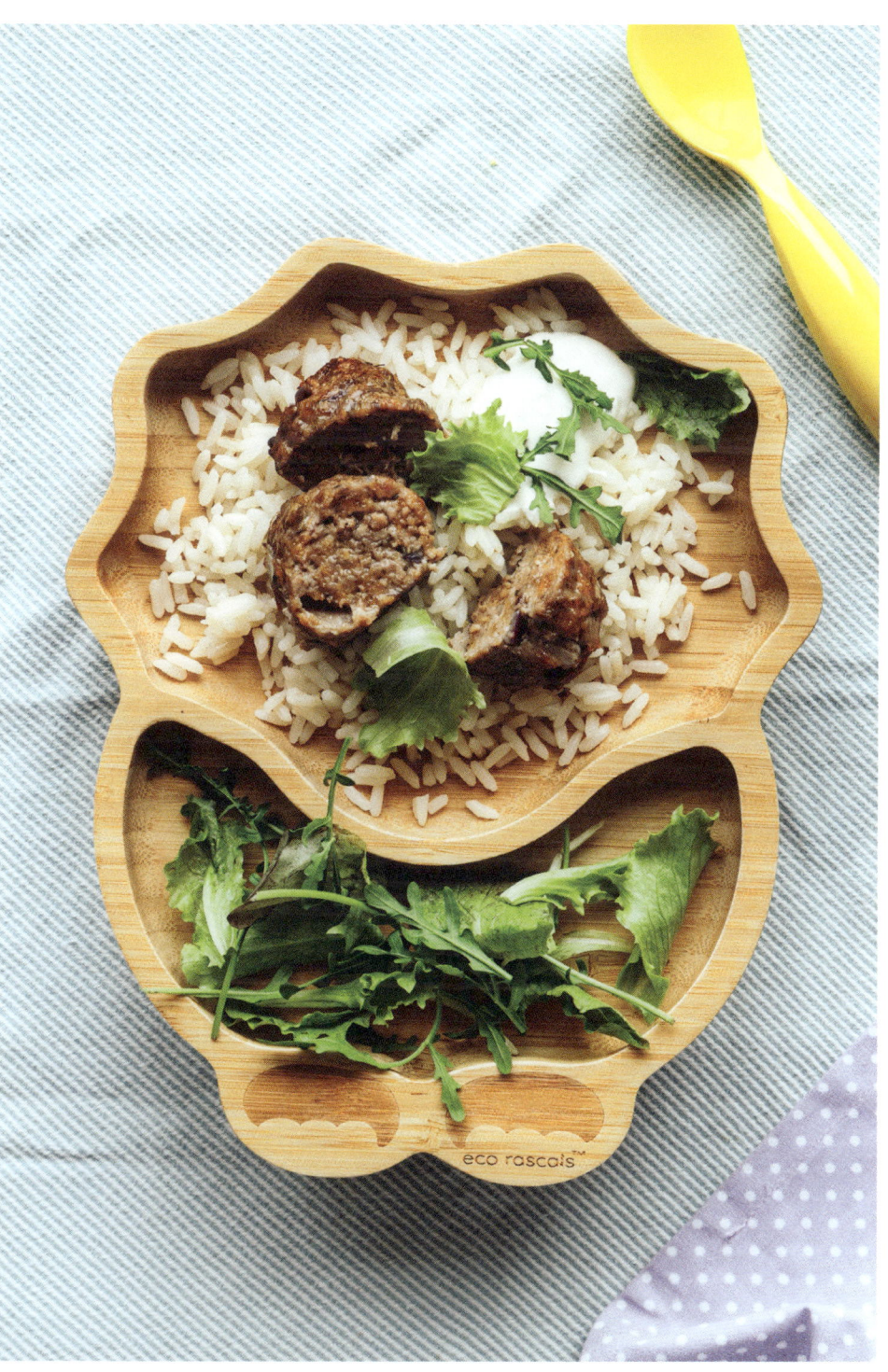

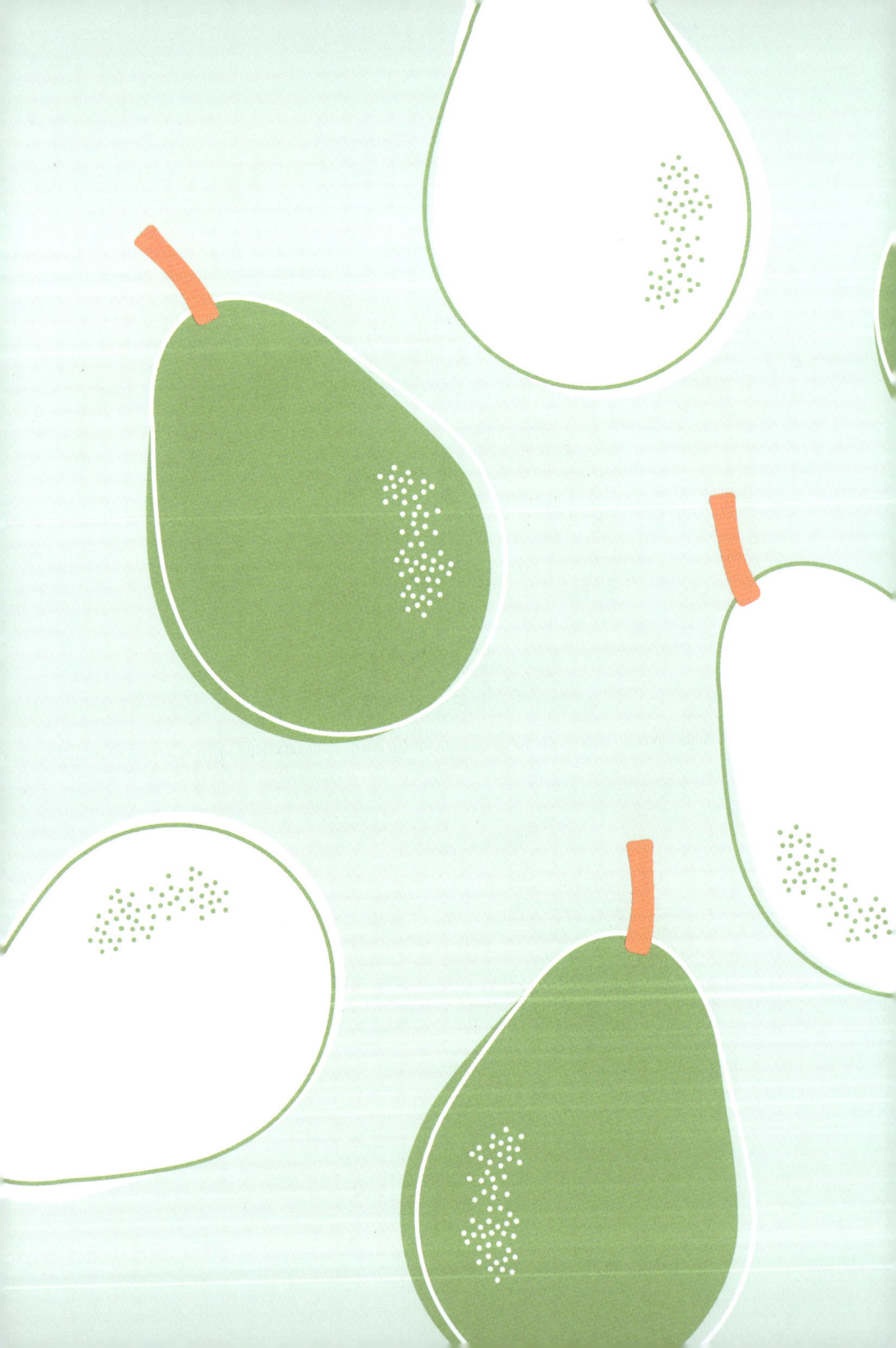

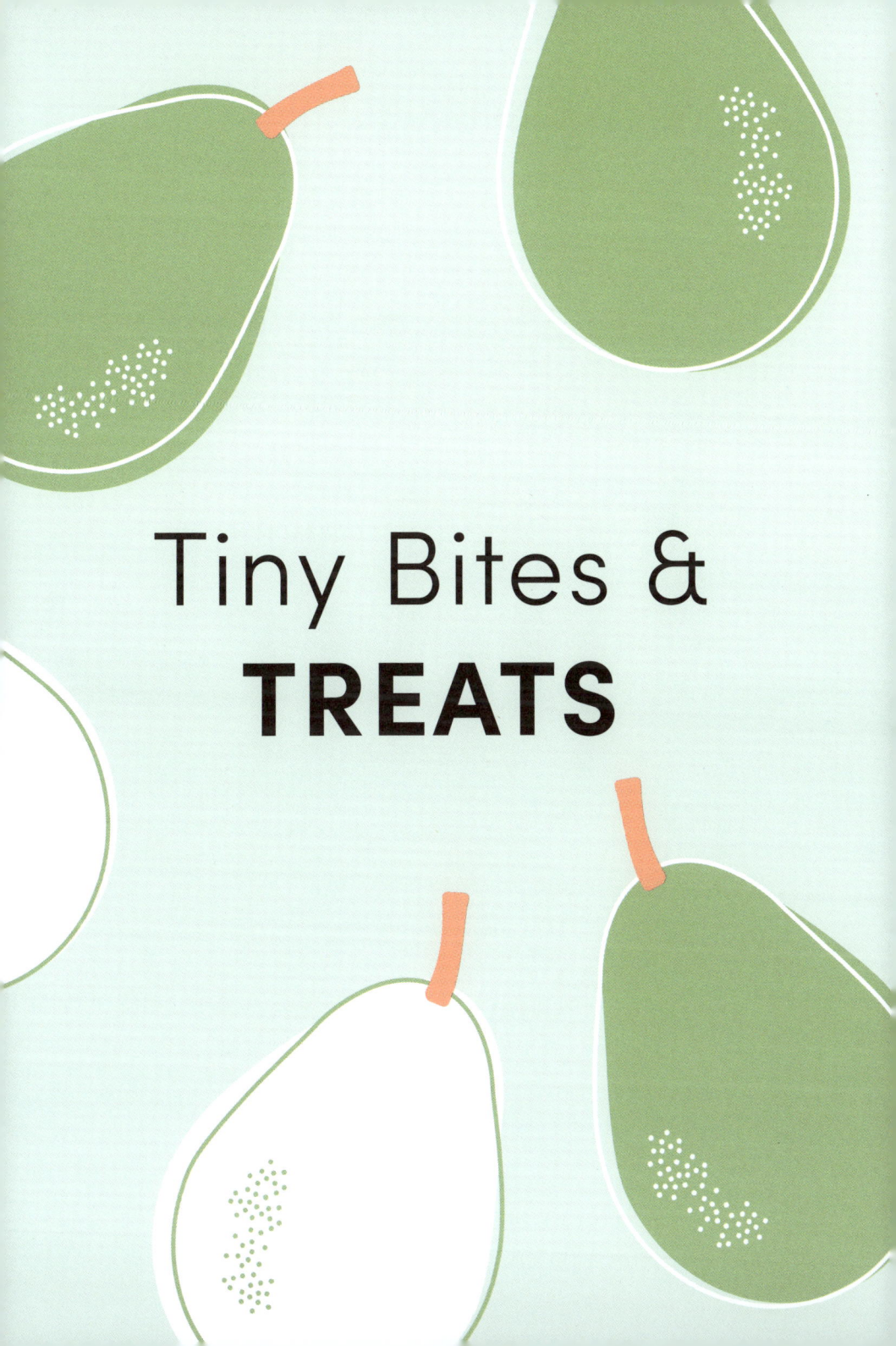

Tiny Bites & **TREATS**

CRISPY PEANUT BALLS

These cold, no-bake crispy peanut balls are perfect for babies struggling with teething – the crunchy chill will help ease those pesky, sore gums. Teething can be as stressful for parents as it is for babies, so have fun crushing those rice cakes to relieve some tension.

Prep time: **20 mins**

MAKES 11 PORTIONS

125g (4½oz/½ cup) smooth peanut butter
2 tablespoons maple syrup or fruit purée
1 teaspoon vanilla extract
4 plain rice cakes, smashed into small crumbs

See image overleaf

1. Place all the ingredients into a bowl and stir well to combine.
2. Take heaped tablespoons of the mix and roll into balls.
3. Place the balls on a tray and transfer to the refrigerator to set for at least 20 minutes, or until they are ready to be enjoyed.
4. Serve in thin matchsticks to safely avoid your baby putting large chunks into their mouth at one time.

Allergy swaps: For a peanut allergy, swap the peanut butter for sunflower butter or tahini.

BERRY BLISS BALLS

||||||||||||||||||||||||||||||||||||||||||||||||||||||||||||||||||||||||||||||||||||||||

Soft, nutritious bites with a delightful blend of ripe strawberries, wholesome oats, sweet ground almonds and a touch of coconut. Watch your baby discover the joy of real food, one blissful bite at a time, with this mess-free, baby-approved snack that encourages self-feeding while also nurturing the tastebuds.

Prep + cook time: **20 mins**

MAKES 11 PORTIONS

175g (6oz/generous
  1 cup) fresh berries
180g (6½oz/2 cups) oats
35g (1¼oz/⅓ cup)
  desiccated (dried
  shredded) coconut, plus
  extra for dusting
30g (1oz/⅓ cup) ground
  almonds
4 tablespoons maple
  syrup (optional)

See image overleaf

1. Place the berries, 45g (1½oz/½ cup) oats, coconut, ground almonds and maple syrup (if using) into a food processor and blend until smooth.
2. Scoop the mixture into a mixing bowl and stir through the remaining oats.
3. Take heaped tablespoons of the mixture and roll it into balls, then roll in more coconut.
4. Place the balls on a tray and transfer to the refrigerator to set for at least 20 minutes, or until they are ready to be enjoyed!
5. Serve in thin matchsticks to safely avoid your baby putting large chunks into their mouth at one time

Allergy swaps: For a nut allergy, swap the ground almonds with an extra 4 tablespoons oats. For a gluten intolerance, use gluten-free oats.

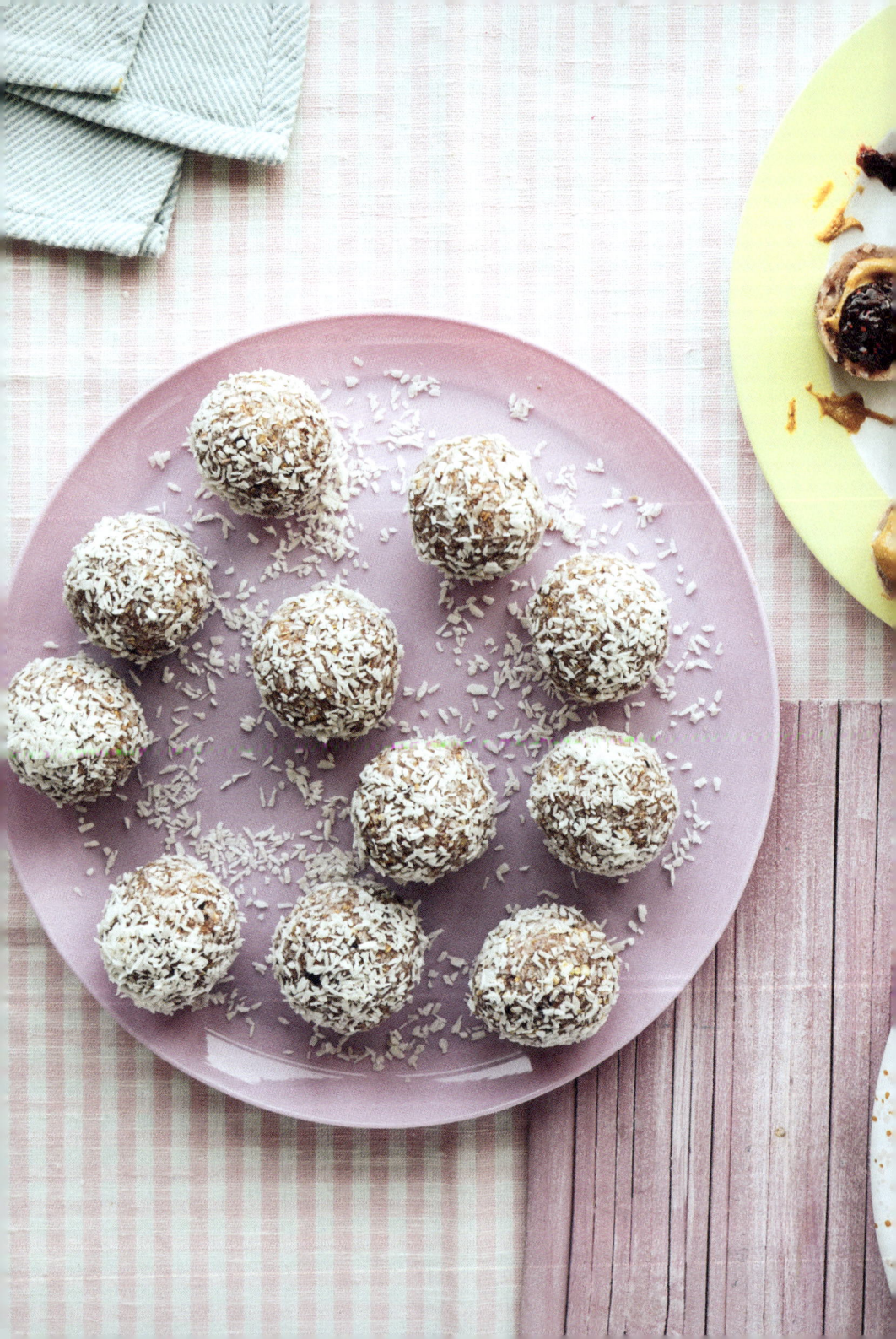

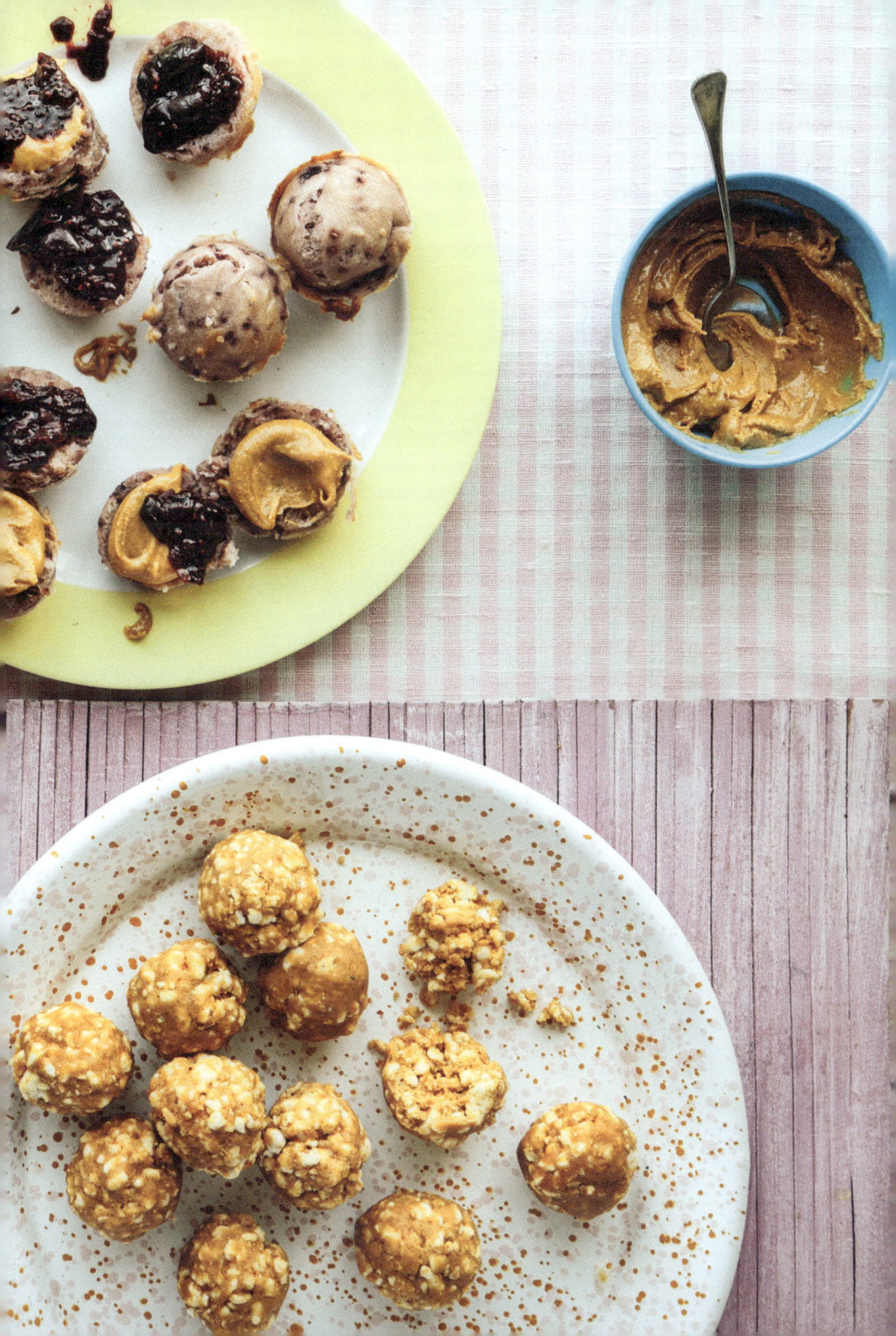

COCONUT AND CHERRY BITES

||||||||||||||||||||||||||||||||||||||||||||||||||||||||||||||||||||||||||||||||||||||||||||||||||

These soft, melt-in-the-mouth delights are crafted with creamy Greek yoghurt, coconut and a hint of sweet strawberry jam. These tropical bites are particularly delicious sliced in half and spread with some low-sugar jam and/or smooth peanut butter.

Prep + cook time: **20 mins**

MAKES 24 PORTIONS

420g (15oz/3½ cups)
  self-raising
  (self-rising) flour
450ml (15fl oz/scant
  2 cups) coconut-style
  Greek yoghurt
5 tablespoons Homemade
  Fruity Jam made with
  cherries (see page 100)
  or use shop-bought
  low-sugar cherry jam
5 tablespoons desiccated
  (dried shredded)
  coconut
2 tablespoons maple
  syrup (optional)

See image on previous
  page

1. Preheat the oven to 210°C/190°C fan/425°F/Gas mark 7 and grease a 24-hole mini-muffin tray or line with muffin cases.
2. Combine all the ingredients in a food processor and pulse until the mixture comes together.
3. Divide the mixture evenly between the prepared muffin holes or cases, then cook in the oven for 15 minutes, or until slightly golden and a knife inserted into the centre comes out clean.
4. Serve once cooled.

Allergy swaps: For a dairy allergy, swap the yoghurt for a soya or oat alternative with 1 teaspoon coconut extract stirred in. For a gluten intolerance, swap the flour for a gluten-free variety.

EASY NO-SUGAR BISCUITS

My simple and wholesome no-sugar biscuits (cookies) are perfect for little hands. Not only do these treats offer a delightful taste experience for your little one, but they also provide a range of essential nutrients to support their growth and development, such as fibre, protein, calcium and vitamin E.

Prep + cook time: **20 mins**

MAKES 8 PORTIONS

1 x 90g (3oz/generous ⅓ cup) apple fruit purée pouch
2 tablespoons smooth peanut butter
165g (6oz/1⅔ cups) ground almonds
2 tablespoons whole (full-fat) milk

1. Preheat the oven to 180°C/160°C fan/350°F/Gas mark 4, and line a large baking tray (sheet pan) with baking parchment.
2. Place the ingredients in a mixing bowl and stir well to form a thick dough.
3. Roll the dough out to a 5mm (¼in) thickness and cut it into small cookies using a 6cm (2¼in) cookie cutter.
4. Place the cookies on the prepared baking tray and bake for 12–15 minutes until golden. Alternatively, air-fry at 140°C/285°F for 12 minutes.
5. Serve once cooled.

Allergy swaps: For a dairy allergy, swap the milk for soya, oat, coconut, breast or formula milk. For a peanut allergy, swap the peanut butter for sunflower butter or tahini. For a nut allergy, swap the almonds for ground oats.

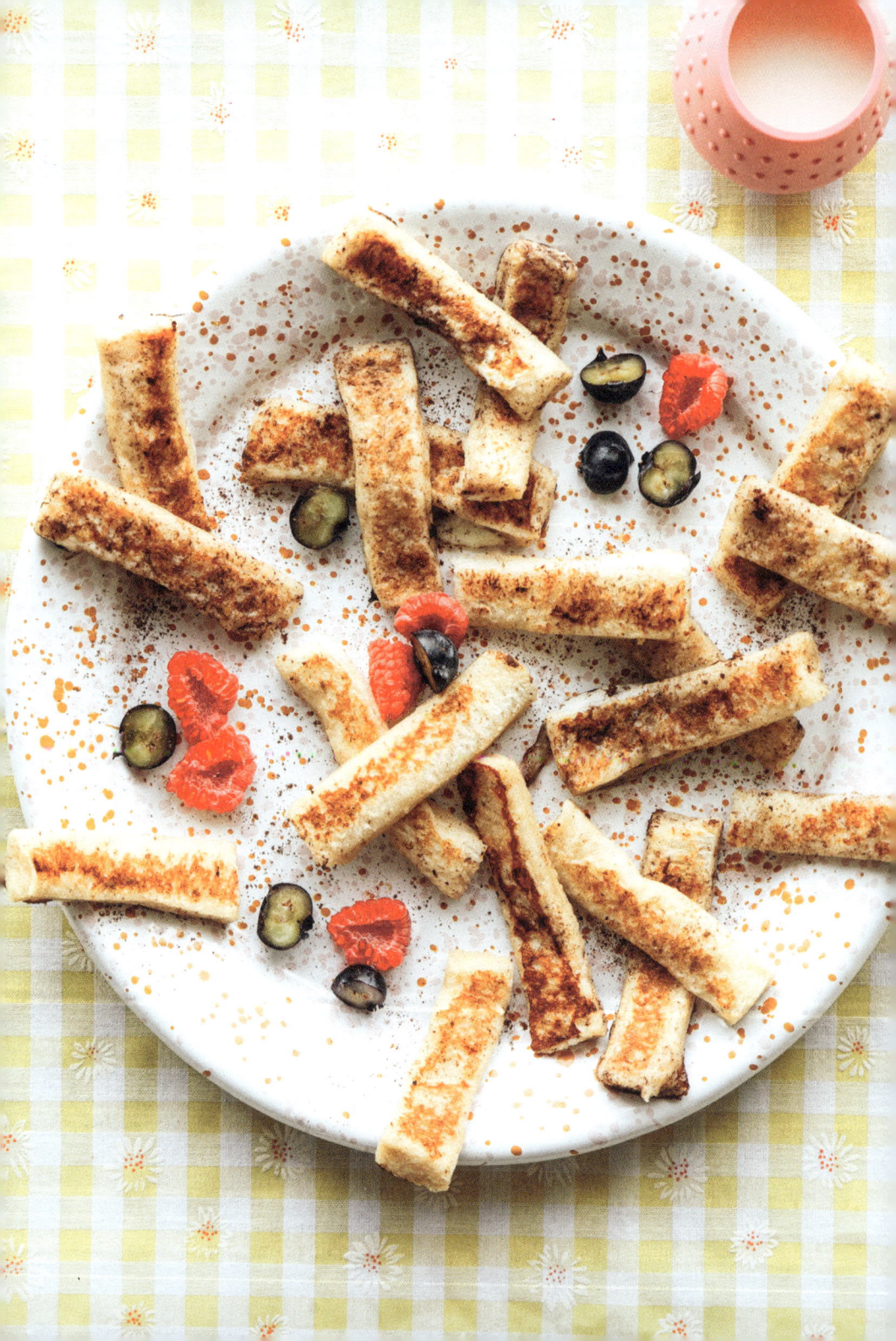

CRISPY CINNAMON STICKS

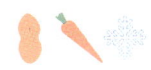

These delectable cinnamon sticks are an irresistible blend of sweetness and spice. With a crispy coating and soft, fluffy centre, they are the epitome of indulgence. Plus, they're freezer-friendly and can be defrosted in 15 minutes, making them an essential for busy parents.

Prep + cook time: **15 mins**

MAKES 4 PORTIONS

125ml (4¼fl oz/½ cup) whole (full-fat) milk
1 medium egg
60ml (2fl oz/¼ cup) maple syrup or fruit purée
1½ teaspoons ground cinnamon, plus extra for sprinkling
1½ teaspoons vanilla extract
4 slices white bread, cut into finger-width batons
1 tablespoon unsalted butter

1. Put the milk, egg, maple syrup, cinnamon and vanilla extract into a jug (pitcher) and whisk well.
2. Pour the mix into a shallow bowl and add half of the bread pieces. Let the bread soak up the eggy mixture for 1–2 minutes.
3. Heat the butter in a large frying pan (skillet) over a medium heat. Once melted, add the eggy bread and fry the slices for 2 minutes on each side until golden. As the first batch fries, add the second batch to soak in the egg.
4. Once the first batch is cooked, transfer it to a plate, cover with tin foil to keep warm and fry the second batch in the same way until golden and crisp.
5. Dust with an extra sprinkling of cinnamon, allow to cool and enjoy!

Allergy swaps: For a dairy allergy, swap the milk for soya, oat, coconut, breast or formula milk, and swap the butter for vegetable oil. For an egg allergy, swap the egg for 1 tablespoon ground flaxseed stirred into 3 tablespoons water. For a gluten intolerance, swap the bread for a gluten-free variety.

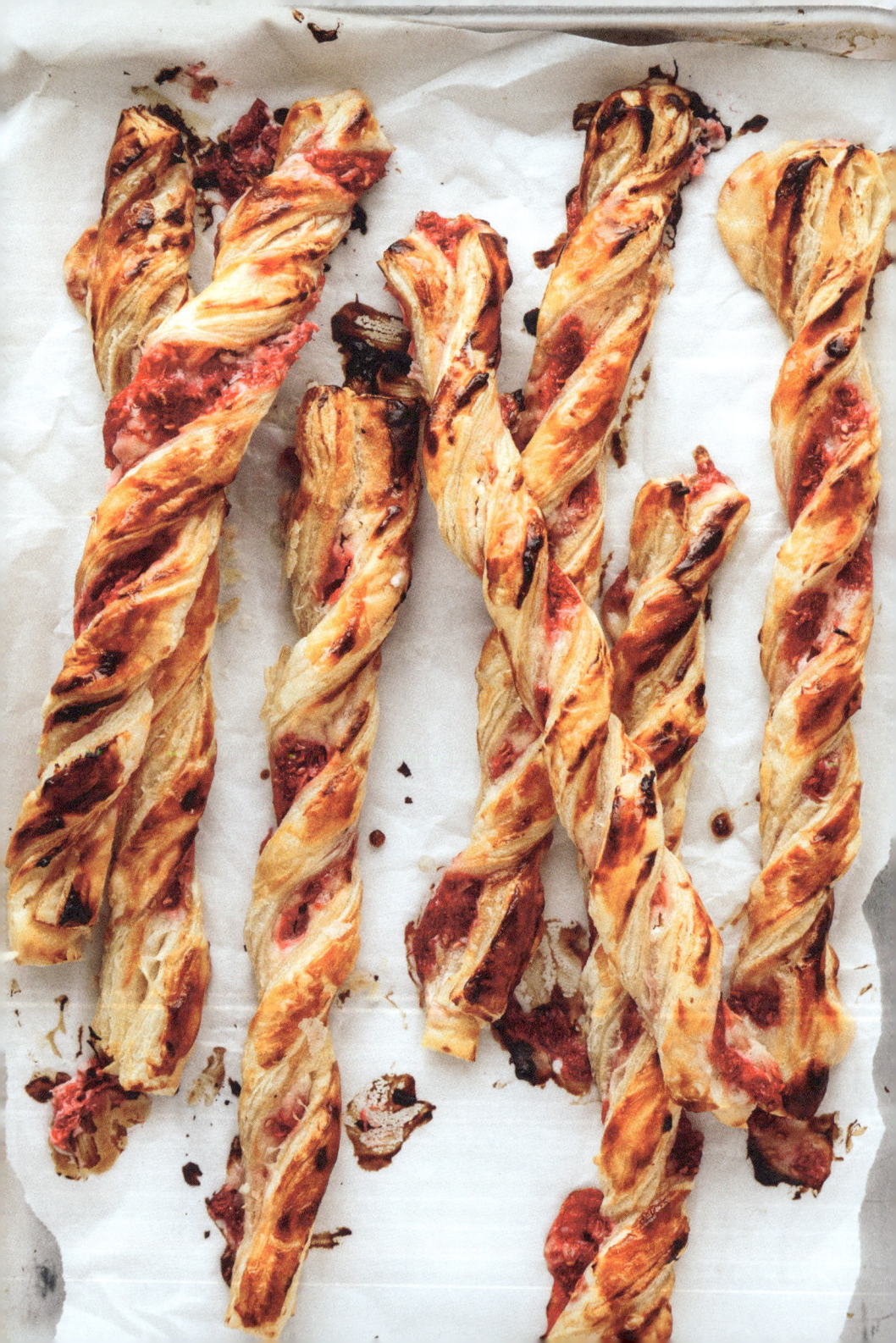

RASPBERRY AND LEMON CHEESECAKE TWISTS

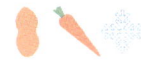

|||||||||||||||||||||||||||||||||||||||||||||||||||||||||||||||||||||||||||||||||||||

Crisp, flaky pastry, smooth cream cheese and the tart acidity of raspberries and lemon are a match made in heaven and a gentle way to introduce some sour flavour into your baby's diet. If the lemon is too tart for their liking, you can leave it out, while the raspberries can be swapped for any berry you desire.

Prep + cook time: **20 mins**

MAKES 10 PORTIONS

5 tablespoons cream cheese
2 tablespoons lemon curd
1 ready-rolled puff pastry sheet
60g (2oz/½ cup) raspberries, mashed
1 small egg, beaten

1. Preheat the oven to 200°C/180°C fan/400°F/Gas mark 6, and line a large baking tray (sheet pan) with baking parchment.
2. In a small bowl, mix together the cream cheese and lemon curd until well combined.
3. Unroll the puff pastry sheet horizontally and coat one half with the cream cheese mix. Spoon the mashed raspberries evenly over the cream cheese.
4. Fold the uncoated pastry over the coated pastry.
5. Cut the pastry into 10 x 1cm (½in) strips. I like to use a pizza cutter for this step.
6. Twist the strips 3 or 4 times, then place them onto the prepared baking tray. Brush with egg wash, then bake the twists in the oven for 15 minutes, or until golden brown. Alternatively, air-fry at 160°C/325°F for 12 minutes.
7. Serve once cooled.

   Allergy swaps: Swap the cream cheese for a dairy-free soft cheese. For an egg allergy, swap the egg for 2 teaspoons milk or vegetable oil. For a gluten intolerance, swap the puff pastry for gluten-free.

MINI GREEN MONSTER MUFFINS

IIIIIIIIIIIIIIIIIIIIIIIIIIIIIIIIIIIIIIIIIIIIIIIIIIIIIIIIIIIIIIIIIIIIIIIIIIIIIIIIIIIIIIIIIIIIIIIIIIIIIIIIIIIIIIIIIIIIIII

Mini green monster muffins are a powerhouse of flavour and nutrition, bursting with nourishing ingredients such as oats, bananas, spinach and Greek yoghurt.

Prep + cook time: 20 mins

MAKES 12 PORTIONS

240g (8½oz/2 cups)
  self-raising
  (self-rising) flour
45g (1½oz/½ cup) oats
1 large banana
3 handfuls of spinach
185ml (6¼fl oz/¾ cup)
  full-fat Greek yoghurt
60ml (2fl oz/¼ cup) maple
  syrup or fruit purée
2 medium eggs
1 teaspoon vanilla extract

1. Preheat the oven to 180°C/160°C fan/350°F/Gas mark 4, and grease a 12-hole mini-muffin tray or line with muffin cases.
2. Put all of the ingredients into a food processor and blend to create a smooth batter.
3. Divide the mixture evenly between your prepared mini-muffin cups and place into the oven for 15 minutes, or until slightly golden and a knife inserted into the centre comes out clean.
4. Serve once cooled.

Allergy swaps: For a dairy allergy, swap the yoghurt for a soya, coconut or oat alternative. For an egg allergy, swap the eggs for 2 tablespoons ground flaxseed stirred into 6 tablespoons water. For a gluten intolerance, swap the flour for a gluten-free variety.

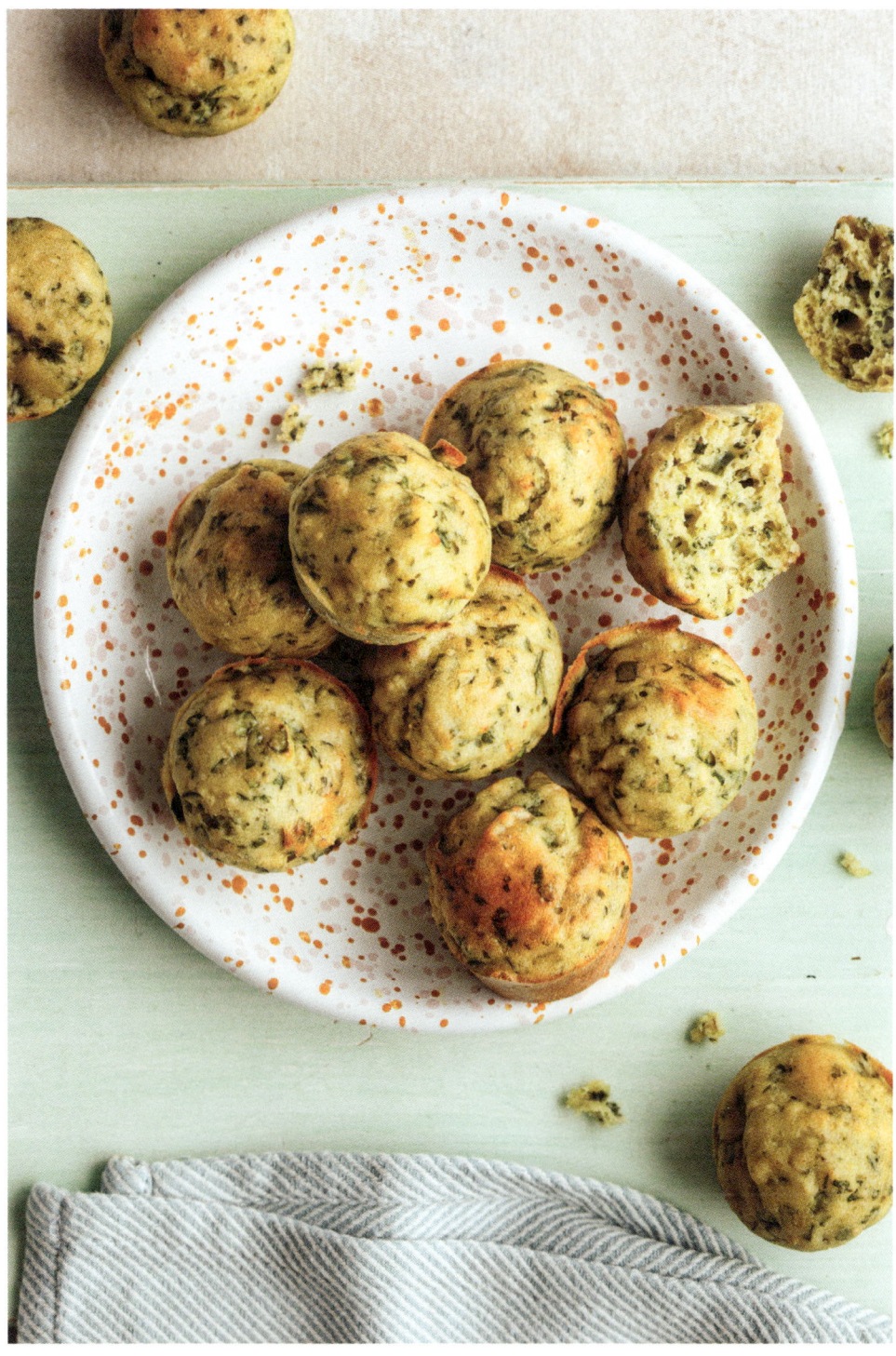

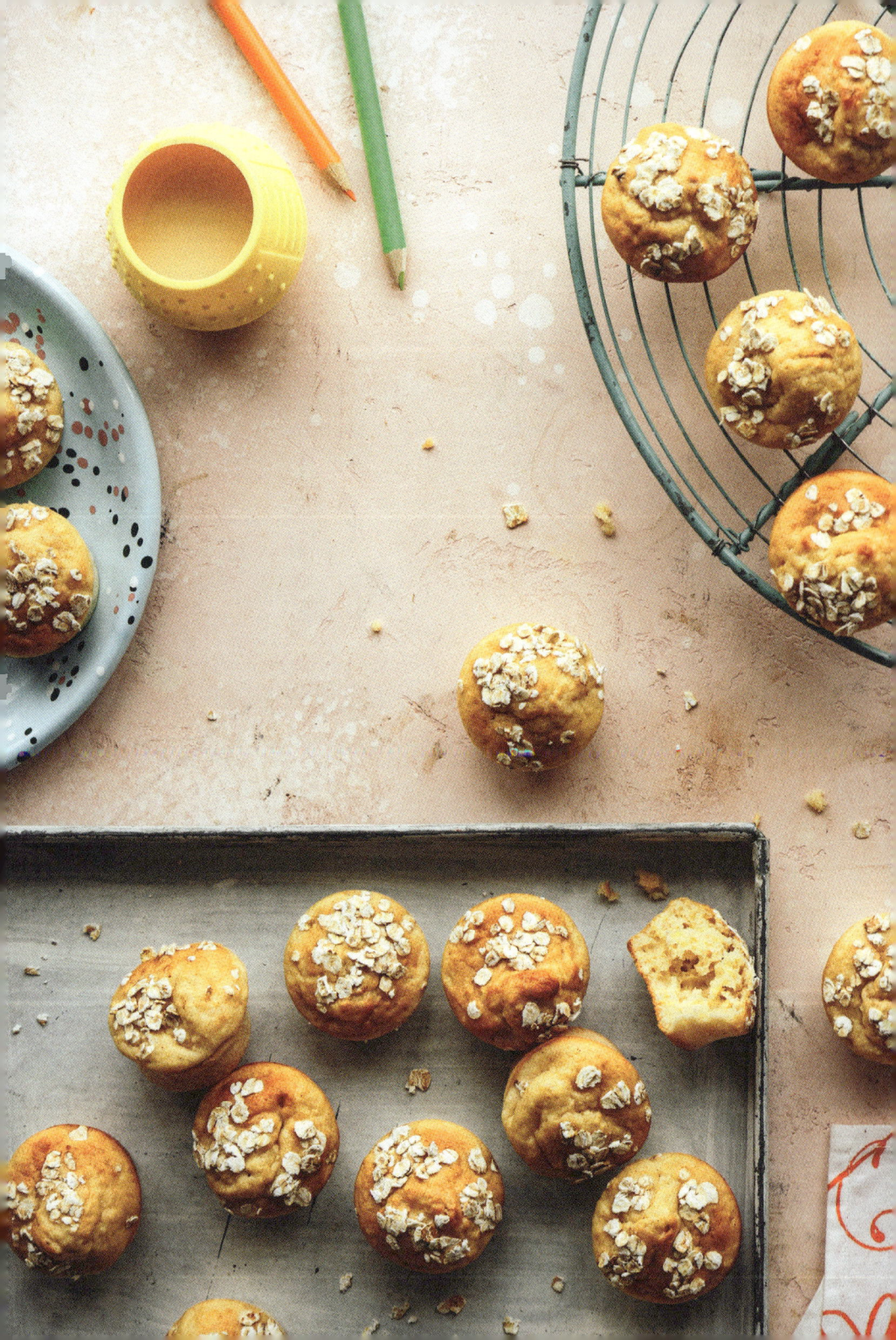

APPLE, PEAR AND CINNAMON MINI MUFFINS

My kids love making these 'throw-it-all-in' mini muffins with me. They watch, fascinated, as the ingredients whizz up, before miraculously turning into delicious little cakes before their very eyes. Ideal for stocking up your freezer stash with minimal effort.

Prep + cook time: **20 mins**

MAKES 24 PORTIONS

1 apple, peeled and
   roughly diced
1 pear, peeled and
   roughly diced
2 medium eggs
80ml (2¾fl oz/⅓ cup)
   whole (full-fat) milk
80ml (2¾fl oz/⅓ cup)
   maple syrup or
   fruit purée
180g (6½oz/1½ cups)
   self-raising
   (self-rising) flour
oats, for sprinkling
   (optional)

1. Preheat the oven to 200°C/180°C fan/400°F/Gas mark 6, and grease a 24-hole mini-muffin tray or line with muffin cases.
2. Put all of the ingredients, except the oats, into a food processor and blend to create a smooth batter.
3. Divide the mixture evenly between your prepared mini-muffin cups, sprinkle with oats (if using) and place in the oven for 15 minutes, or until golden and a knife inserted in the centre comes out clean.
4. Serve once cooled.

Allergy swaps: For a dairy allergy, swap the milk for soya, oat, coconut, breast or formula milk. For an egg allergy, swap the eggs for 2 tablespoons ground flaxseed stirred into 6 tablespoons water. For a gluten intolerance, swap the flour for a gluten-free variety.

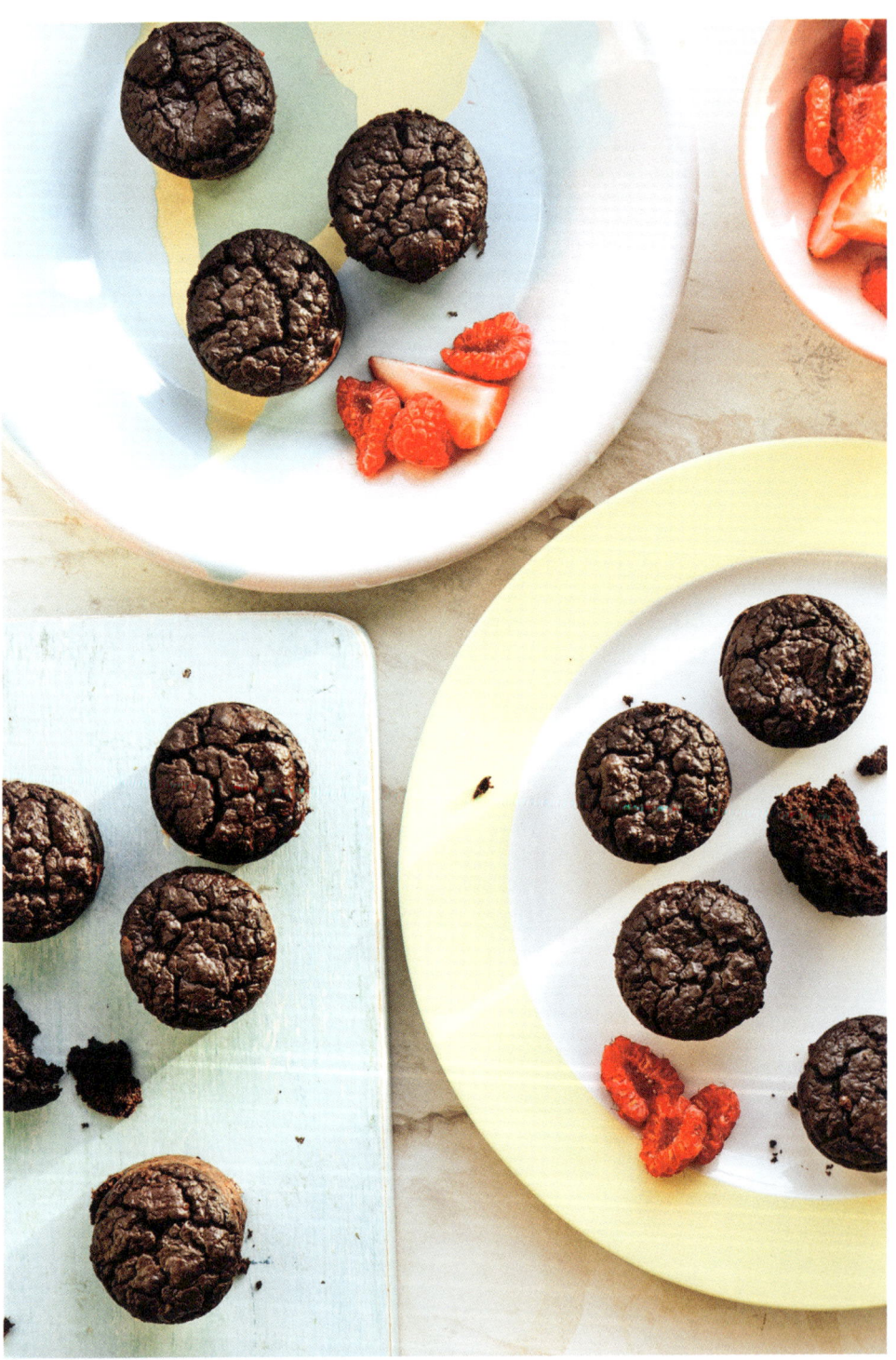

MINI BROWNIE BITES

These mini brownies are a win-win for parents and little ones, with wholesome fun in every bite! Moist, chocolatey and irresistibly gooey, there's also a dose of fruity pear goodness, making snack time both delicious and nutritious. Perfectly sized for lunchboxes and picnics.

Prep + cook time: **15 mins**

MAKES 12 PORTIONS

2 pears, peeled, cored
   and roughly diced
2 medium eggs
2 tablespoons peanut
   butter
1 teaspoon baking
   powder
50g (1¾oz/½ cup) cocoa
   powder (for a less bitter
   taste, opt for a low-
   sugar hot chocolate
   powder instead)

1. Preheat the oven to 200°C/180°C fan/400°F/Gas mark 6, and grease 12 holes of a 24-hole mini-muffin tray.
2. Place all of the ingredients into a food processor and blend until smooth.
3. Spoon the mixture evenly between the mini-muffin tray cups, then place into the oven to bake for 10–12 minutes, or until they turn a rich chocolate brown in colour and a knife inserted into the centre comes out clean.
4. Serve once cooled.

Allergy swaps: For an egg allergy, swap the eggs for 2 tablespoons ground flaxseed stirred into 3 tablespoons water. For a peanut allergy, swap the peanut butter for sunflower butter or tahini.

CINNAMON AND VANILLA DOUGHNUT STICKS

|||||||||||||||||||||||||||||||||||||||||||||||||||||||||||||||||||||||||||||||||||||||||||||||||||||||||||

Easy to handle, and irresistibly soft and fluffy, these dough sticks were developed as a healthier, baby-friendly twist on traditional doughnuts, infused with the warmth of cinnamon and the sweetness of vanilla.

Prep + cook time: **15 mins**

MAKES 7 PORTIONS

50g (1¾oz/½ cup) ground almonds

60g (2oz/½ cup) self-raising (self-rising) flour

3 tablespoons oats

2 tablespoons coconut sugar, plus 1 teaspoon for rolling (optional)

1 medium egg

60ml (2fl oz/¼ cup) vegetable oil

2 teaspoons vanilla extract

3 tablespoons unsalted butter, melted

1 teaspoon ground cinnamon

1. Preheat the oven to 220°C/200°C fan/450°F/Gas mark 7, and line a large baking tray (sheet pan) with baking parchment.
2. Place the ground almonds, flour, oats, sugar (if using), egg, oil and vanilla extract in a large mixing bowl and stir well to combine.
3. Take a tablespoon of the mix at a time and roll into balls. Roll each ball between your hands to make skinny sausages, about 1.5cm (⅔in) thickness.
4. Add the melted butter, cinnamon and 1 teaspoon coconut sugar into a shallow bowl and stir to combine.
5. Dip the dough sticks in the cinnamon butter, then place them onto the prepared baking tray and bake in the oven for 8–10 minutes until golden. Alternatively, bake in an air fryer at 180°C/350°F for 6–8 minutes.
6. Serve once cooled.

Allergy swaps: Swap the butter for a dairy-free alternative. Swap the egg for 60ml (2fl oz/¼ cup) dairy, soya, coconut or oat yoghurt. For a gluten intolerance, swap the flour for a gluten-free variety.

HERBY PARMESAN TORTILLA CHIPS

Elevate your little one's snack game with these family-friendly tortilla chips – a tasty and effortless treat that's healthier and more flavourful than shop-bought. These chips are particularly delicious dipped into garlic and herb cream cheese.

Prep + cook time: **12 mins**

MAKES 3 PORTIONS

3 mini tortilla wraps
1 tablespoon vegetable oil
1 tablespoon grated
  Parmesan cheese
½ teaspoon dried oregano
½ teaspoon dried
  rosemary

1. Preheat the oven to 220°C/200°C fan/450°F/Gas mark 7, and line a large baking tray (sheet pan) with baking parchment.
2. Slice each tortilla like a pizza into 8 tortilla chip-shaped triangles, and place them into a mixing bowl.
3. Add the remaining ingredients and stir to coat the tortillas well.
4. Place the tortilla crisps in a single layer on the prepared baking tray and bake for 6–8 minutes until crispy enough to 'snap'. Alternatively, air-fry at 180°C/350°F for 5 minutes.
5. Serve once cooled.

   Allergy swaps: For a dairy allergy, swap the Parmesan for ½ tablespoon nutritional yeast or 1 tablespoon dairy-free hard cheese. For a gluten intolerance swap the tortilla wraps for a gluten-free variety.

OOZY LAVA STICKS

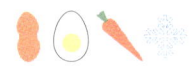

My kids go crazy for these oozy, tortilla-wrapped cheese sticks, perfectly sized for little hands to grasp. And even better, they sneak in some crunchy carrots, adding a dose of vegetable goodness to this delicious treat.

Prep + cook time: **15 mins**

MAKES 8 PORTIONS

240g (8½oz/2 cups) grated Red Leicester cheese
1 carrot, grated
½ teaspoon dried mixed herbs
4 large tortilla wraps
60ml (2fl oz/¼ cup) unsalted butter, melted

1. Preheat the oven to 220°C/200°C fan/450°F/Gas mark 7, and line a large baking tray (sheet pan) with baking parchment.
2. Mix the grated cheese, carrot and mixed herbs together in a bowl.
3. Add a quarter of the mix to one end of each tortilla, then roll them up to wrap the filling tightly.
4. Slice each roll in half and place them onto the prepared baking tray. Brush the sticks with the melted butter and bake for 10 minutes, or until golden and crispy. Alternatively, air-fry at 180°C/350°F for 5 minutes.
5. Serve once cooled.

Allergy swaps: For a dairy allergy, swap the Red Leicester cheese for a dairy-free alternative and swap the butter for vegetable oil. For a gluten intolerance, swap the tortilla wraps for a gluten-free variety.

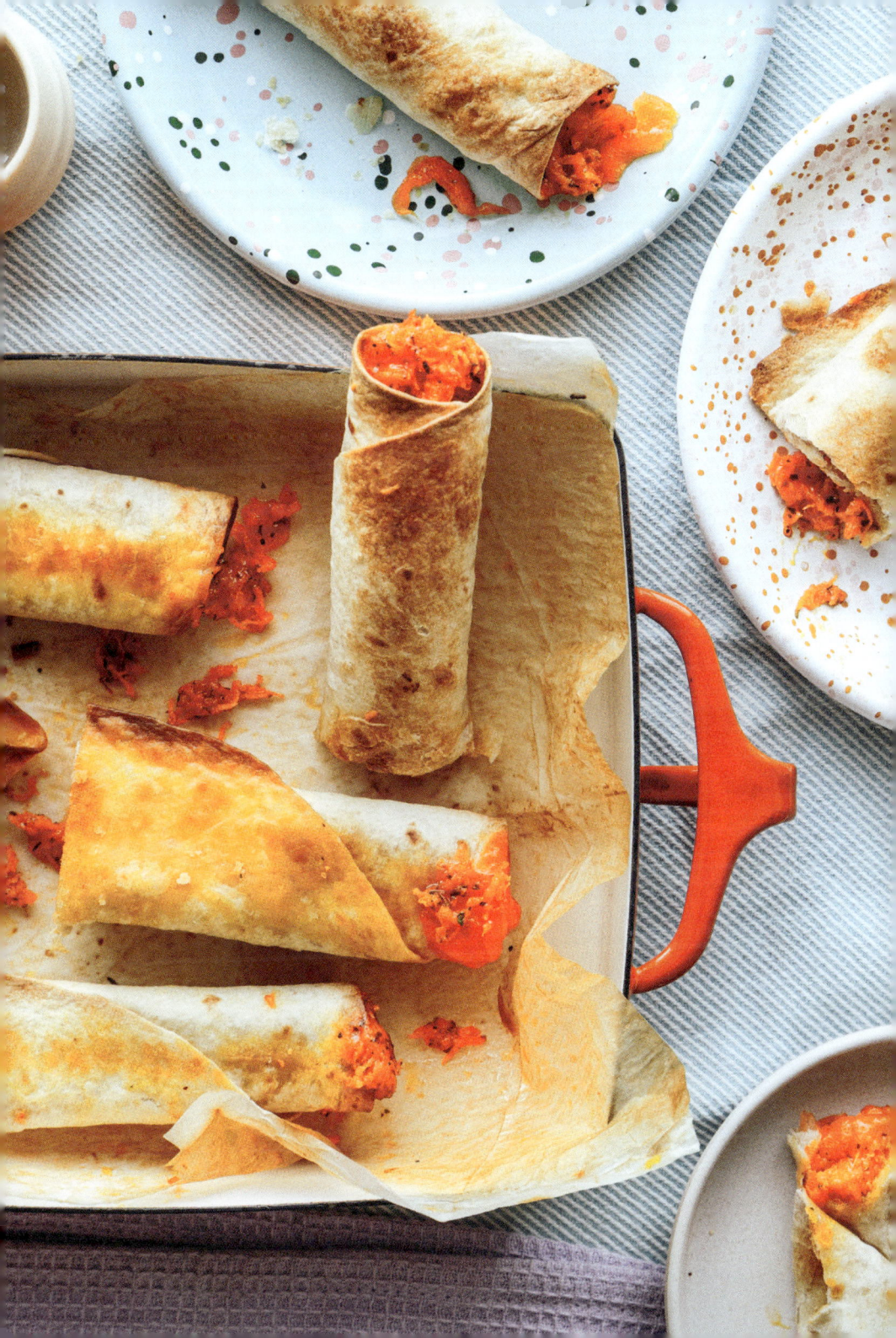

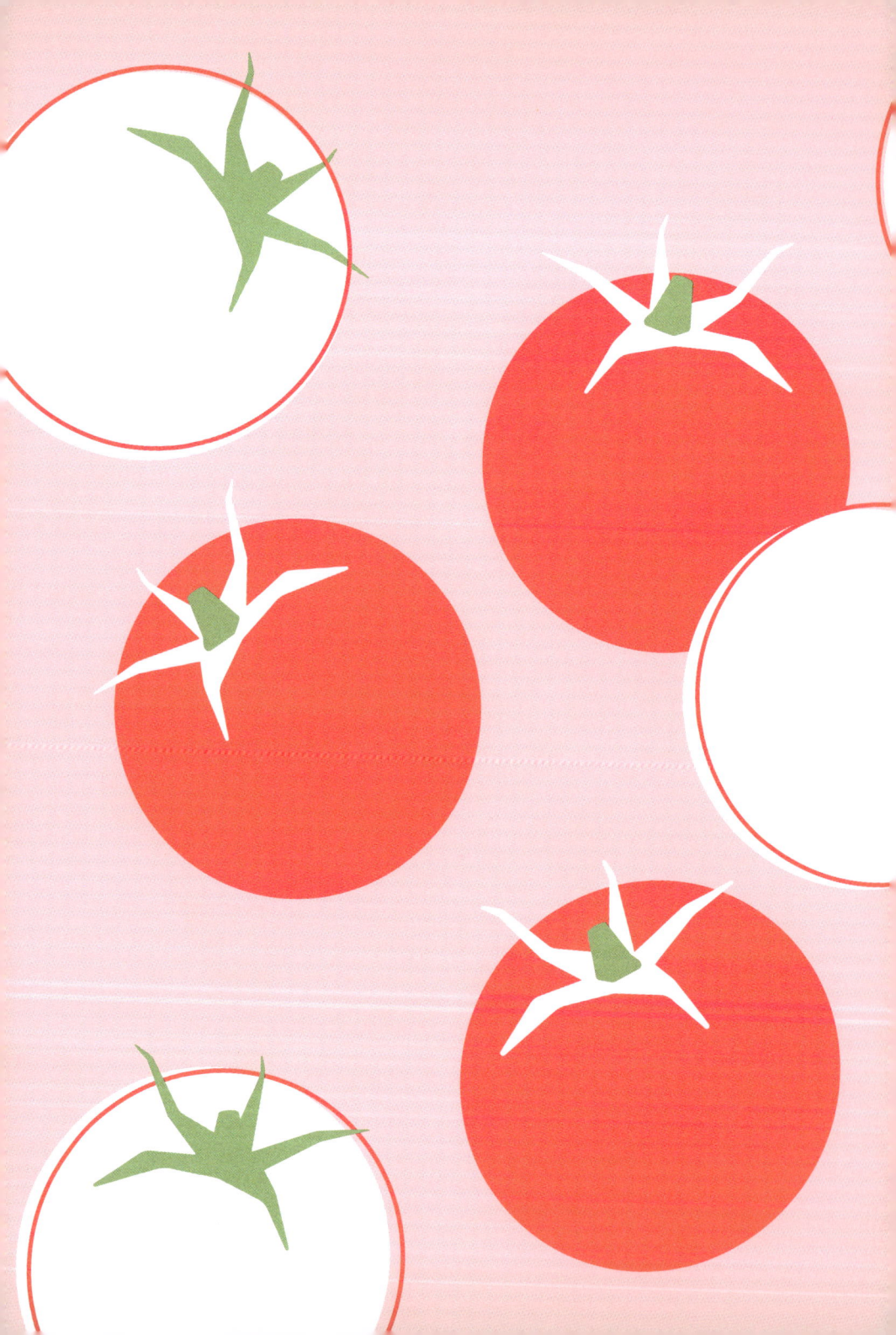

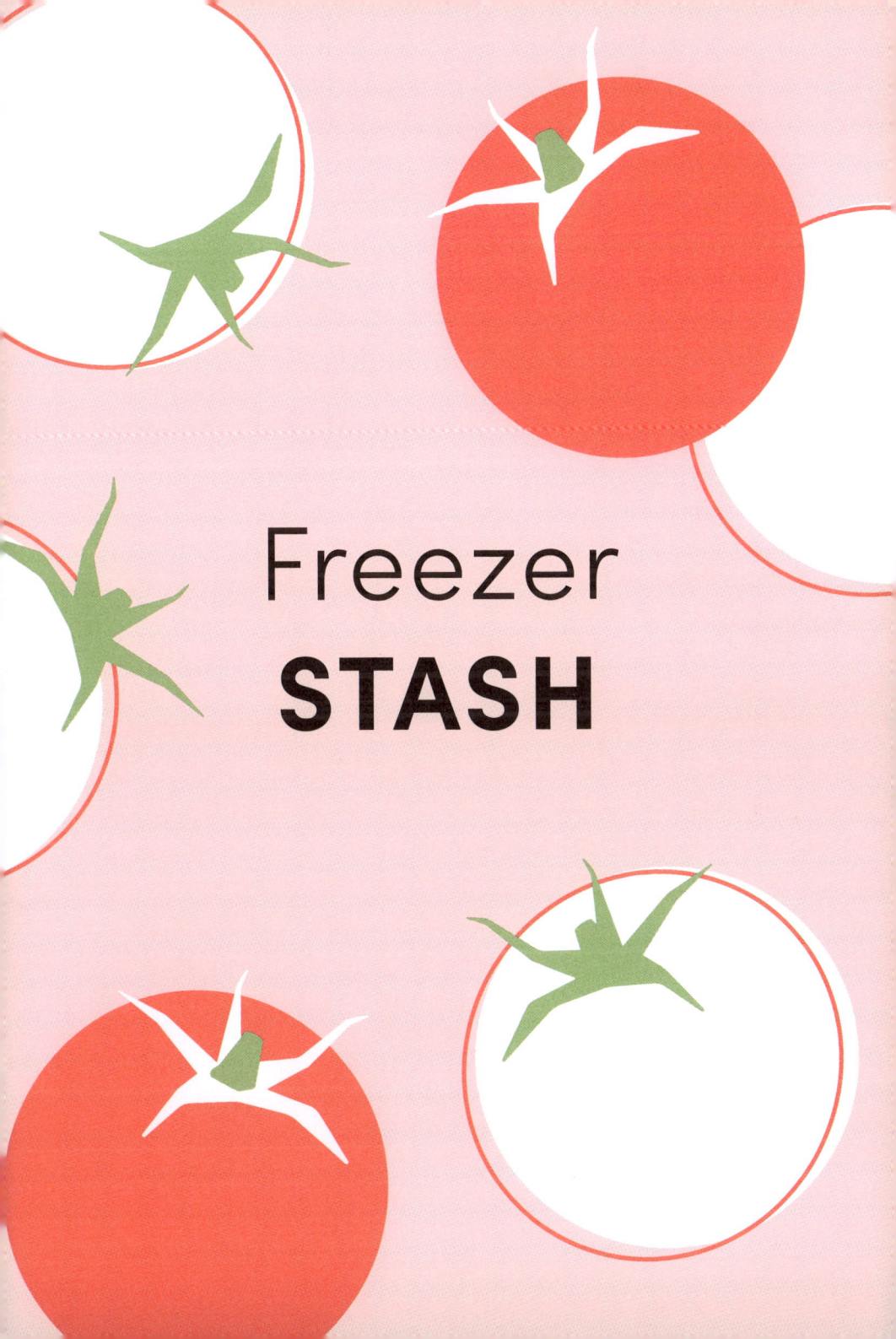

Freezer
STASH

PINK PURÉE CUBES

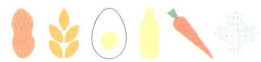

This delicious pink berry purée will add a sweet touch to your baby's porridge or yoghurt. For ultimate convenience, freeze the purée in ice-cube trays, ready to be stirred into warm breakfasts right from the freezer. Feel free to switch things up by swapping the blueberries for any berry of your choice.

Prep + cook time: **10 mins**

MAKES 50+ PORTIONS (depending on the size of the ice-cube tray)

400g (14oz/2½ cups) frozen blueberries
3 tablespoons maple syrup (optional)

1. Place the frozen blueberries and maple syrup (if using) into a saucepan and warm over a medium heat for 5 minutes.
2. After 5 minutes, transfer the blueberry mixture to a food processor or blender and blend to a purée.
3. Leave to cool, then pour into ice-cube trays to freeze.
4. Once the cubes are frozen, after at least 4 hours, remove them from the ice-cube trays and transfer them into freezer bags for storage.

Serving options: Use to naturally sweeten muffins or loaves. Stir frozen cubes into porridge until melted or defrost and add to yoghurts to sweeten.

EASY PESTO ICE CUBES

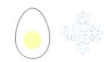

||||||||||||||||||||||||||||||||||||||||||||||||||||||||||||||||||||||||||||||||||||||||||||||||||||||||||||||||

These pesto ice cubes make mealtimes a breeze. When lunch or dinner comes around, just pop a few into a saucepan with freshly cooked pasta and let the vibrant pesto defrost and warm through. It's a hassle-free, flavourful meal that your tiny foodie will love!

Prep time: **5 mins**

MAKES 30+ PORTIONS (depending on the size of the ice-cube tray)

6 teaspoons minced garlic
2 large handfuls of fresh basil
40g (1½oz/½ cup) whole blanched almonds
125ml (4¼fl oz/½ cup) olive oil
3 tablespoons grated Parmesan cheese

1. Add all of the ingredients to a blender or food processor and blend to a smooth, thick sauce.
2. Spoon the pesto into ice-cube trays. Once the cubes are frozen, after at least 4 hours, remove them from the ice-cube trays and transfer them into freezer bags for storage.

To reheat: When you're ready to serve the pesto, add a few cubes to a pan with freshly cooked pasta. Warm over a low heat until the cubes are fully defrosted and warmed through. Add any desired additions, such as cooked meat or tinned tuna. Let the pasta cool before serving.

Allergy swaps: For a dairy allergy, swap the Parmesan for a dairy-free alternative. For a nut allergy, swap the almonds for sesame seeds.

BREAKFAST PANCAKE SLICE

||||||||||||||||||||||||||||||||||||||||||||||||||||||||||||||||||||||||||||||||||||||||||||||||||||||

With this foolproof recipe, you can pour your pancake batter effortlessly into a baking tray (sheet pan) and let your oven do the work. It's a real game-changer because you can slice the pancake into long, perfectly shaped batons, which means you'll have a speedy breakfast option for your baby with virtually no waste. Delicious, convenient and ideal for busy mornings!

Prep + cook time: **20 mins**

MAKES 40+ PORTIONS

500g (1 lb 2oz/4 cups)
  self-raising
  (self-rising) flour
500ml (17fl oz/2 cups)
  whole (full-fat) milk
125ml (½ cup) full-fat
  Greek yoghurt
3 medium eggs
2 teaspoons vanilla
  extract

Allergy swaps: Swap the milk for soya, oat, coconut, breast or formula milk, and swap the yoghurt for a soya, coconut or oat alternative. Swap the eggs for 'vegan' eggs. Swap the flour for gluten-free.

1. Preheat the oven to 200°C/180°C fan/400°F/Gas mark 6, and grease or line a large rimmed baking tray (sheet pan), approximately 43 x 29 x 2cm (17 x 11½ x ¾in), with baking parchment.
2. Place the flour in a mixing bowl.
3. In a jug (pitcher), whisk together the milk, yoghurt, eggs and vanilla extract, then slowly stir the wet mix into the flour to form a smooth batter.
4. Pour the batter into the prepared baking tray and smooth it out with the back of a spoon.
5. Place the tray into the oven to bake for 15 minutes, or until golden. Let the pancake cool completely, then slice into finger-width batons.
6. Place the batons on a baking tray and freeze for up to 1 hour, then transfer to an airtight container or freezer bag and freeze for up to 3 months.

To reheat: Defrost at room temperature for 1 hour, or overnight in the refrigerator. Serve cold, or heat in the microwave for 15 seconds per pancake. Alternatively, you can dry-fry the slices for 1–2 minutes each side, or toast for 60–90 seconds. Let the pancakes cool before serving.

VEGETABLE LOADED PASTA SAUCE

||||||||||||||||||||||||||||||||||||||||||||||||||||||||||||||||||||||||||||||||||||||||||||||||||||||||||||||||

This incredible vegetable-loaded pasta sauce is a freezer essential. In just 20 minutes, you can create a nutrient-packed sauce bursting with flavour and filled with the goodness of red (bell) peppers, courgettes (zucchini) and sweet potatoes. It's so easy to defrost, too, making it a perfect speedy dinner option.

Prep + cook time: **20 mins**

MAKES 8–10 PORTIONS

1 onion, sliced into wedges

3 red (bell) peppers, deseeded and sliced

1 courgette (zucchini), cut into 2.5cm (1in) cubes

2 sweet potatoes, cut into 2.5cm (1in) cubes

3 teaspoons minced garlic

2 teaspoons dried mixed herbs

1 x 400g (14oz) tin of chopped tomatoes

3 tablespoons tomato purée (paste)

1. Preheat the oven to 250°C/230°C fan/480°F/Gas mark 9, and grease or line a large rimmed baking tray (sheet pan), approximately 43 x 29 x 2cm (17 x 11½ x ¾in), with baking parchment.
2. Spread the vegetables evenly over the tray.
3. Add the garlic, herbs, chopped tomatoes and tomato purée and stir gently to combine.
4. Place the tray into the oven to bake for 15 minutes.
5. Remove the tray from the oven, let the vegetables cool slightly, then carefully spoon the mixture into a food processor and blend to a smooth sauce (you may need to do this in two batches).
6. Let the sauce cool, then portion it into a large ice-cube tray and freeze
7. Once the cubes are frozen, remove them from the ice-cube trays and transfer them into freezer bags for storage and freeze for up to 3 months.

To reheat: Add a few cubes to a pan with freshly cooked pasta. Warm over a low heat until the cubes are fully defrosted and warmed through. Add any desired additions, such as cooked meat or tinned tuna. Let the pasta cool before serving.

EASY VEGGIE CHILLI

||||||||||||||||||||||||||||||||||||||||||||||||||||||||||||||||||||||||||||||||||||||||||||||||||

My freezer stash never lacks a chilli; it's a must-have staple in my home. This easy veggie version is packed with wholesome goodness from green lentils, kidney beans and juicy tomatoes – the perfect combination of flavour, nutrition and convenience. Serve with rice, potatoes or bread.

Prep + cook time: **20 mins**

MAKES 8–10 PORTIONS

1 teaspoon vegetable oil
2 onions, finely diced
2 red (bell) peppers,
   deseeded and thinly
   sliced
2 teaspoons mild chilli
   powder
2 teaspoons dried oregano
2 x 400g (14oz) tin of
   green lentils, drained
   and rinsed
2 x 400g (14oz) tin of
   kidney beans, mashed
   slightly
4 x 400g (14oz) tin of
   chopped tomatoes
3 tablespoons tomato
   purée (paste)
4 tablespoons low sugar
   and salt tomato ketchup

1. Heat the oil in a large saucepan over a high heat, and fry the onion and red pepper for 3 minutes until softened.
2. Add all of the remaining ingredients, reduce the heat to a simmer and cook for 12 minutes.
3. Let the chilli cool, then portion it into large ice-cube trays or freezer-safe containers and freeze for up to 3 months.

To reheat: When you're ready to serve the chilli, pop as many cubes as needed into a saucepan and warm over a low-medium heat until fully defrosted and piping hot. Let the chilli cool before serving.

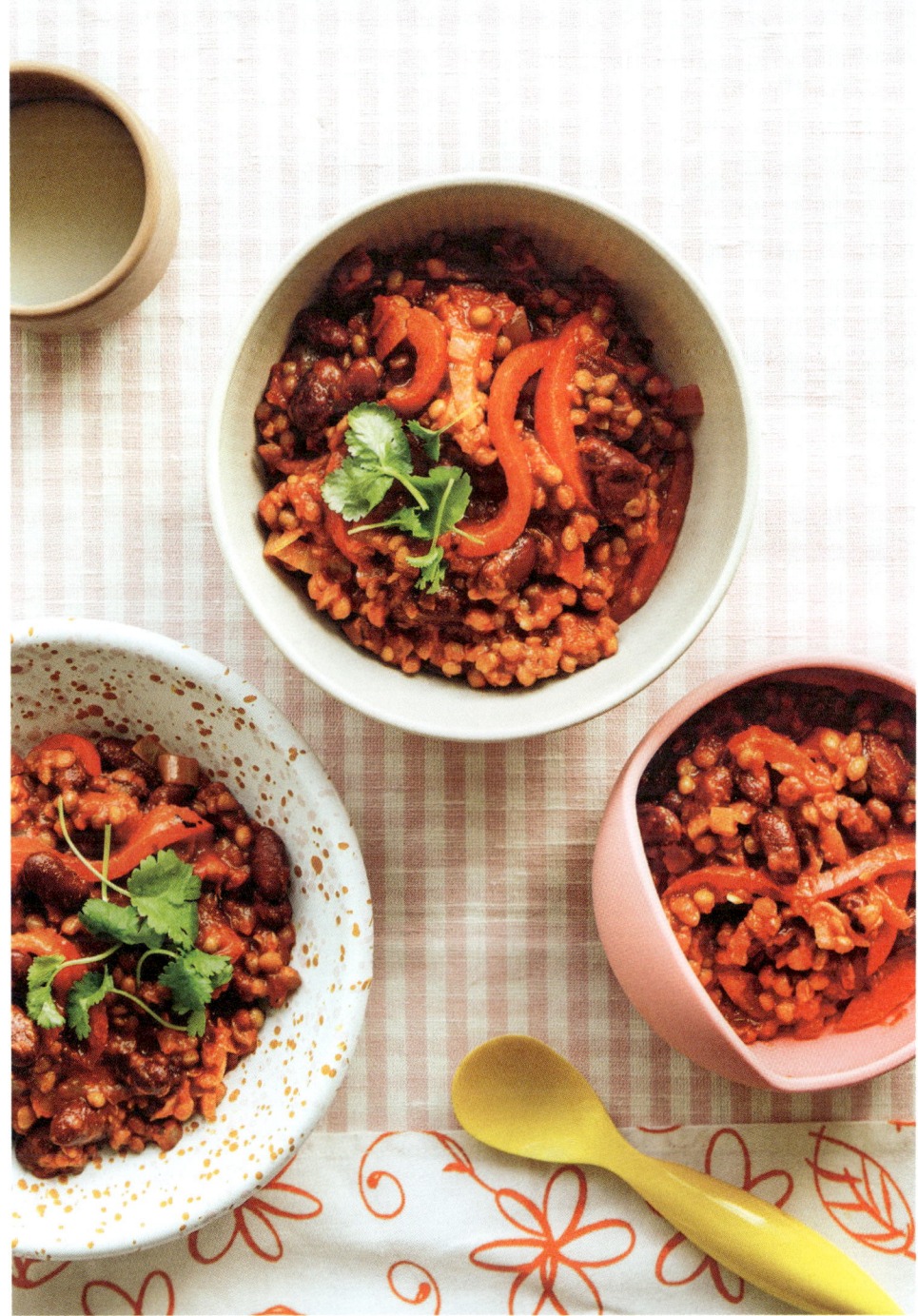

BIG BATCH MUSHROOM AND CARROT BOLOGNESE

||||||||||||||||||||||||||||||||||||||||||||||||||||||||||||||||||||||||||||||||||||||||||

This wholesome, vegetable-packed Bolognese is full of flavour and goodness. It freezes well and is perfect for an easy, midweek family meal.

Prep + cook time: **20 mins**

MAKES 8–10 PORTIONS

2 teaspoons vegetable oil
1 onion, very finely diced
3 carrots, very finely diced
2 teaspoons minced garlic
200g (7oz/2 cups) mushrooms, finely diced
2 teaspoons dried oregano
2 teaspoons dried mixed herbs
2 x 400g (14oz) tins of chopped tomatoes
190g (6¾oz) jar of tomato pesto (you may prefer to use vegan pesto as it is usually lower in salt, but please check the label and pick the best option available)

1. Heat the oil in a large saucepan over a medium heat and fry the onion and carrots for 3 minutes until softened.
2. Add the garlic and mushrooms, stirring consistently for 2 minutes.
3. Add the oregano, mixed herbs, chopped tomatoes and pesto and cover the dish. Cook over a high heat for 10 minutes.
4. Let the Bolognese cool, then portion it into large ice-cube trays or freezer-safe containers and freeze for up to 3 months.

To reheat: Defrost overnight in the refrigerator or reheat directly from frozen. Once you're ready to serve, add the defrosted or still frozen Bolognese to a saucepan and warm over a low-medium heat until fully defrosted and piping hot. Let the Bolognese cool before serving with freshly cooked pasta or spaghetti.

Allergy swaps: For a dairy allergy, swap the pesto for a vegan alternative.

SIMPLE RAGÙ

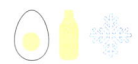

|||||||||||||||||||||||||||||||||||||||||||||||||||||||||||||||||||||||||||||||||||||||||||||||||||||||

A comforting and wholesome ragù, and a favourite among my little ones. Versatile and delicious, it's the ideal companion for pasta, rice, jacket potatoes, or even some simple toast soldiers.

Prep + cook time: **20 mins**

MAKES 8–10 PORTIONS

1 teaspoon olive oil
1 carrot, very finely diced
1 onion, very finely diced
1 stalk of celery, very finely diced
500g (1lb 2oz/generous 2 cups) minced (ground) beef
600ml (20fl oz/2½ cups) passata
400ml (14fl oz/1¾ cups) low-salt beef stock (broth)
2 teaspoons mixed herbs
4 tablespoons low-salt gravy granules

1. Heat the oil in a large saucepan over a high heat, and fry the carrot, onion and celery for 3 minutes until softened.
2. Add the minced beef and fry for 5 minutes until cooked through and browned.
3. Add all of the remaining ingredients and cook over a high heat for 10 minutes (see Note).
4. Let the ragù cool, then portion it into large ice-cube trays or freezer-safe containers and freeze for up to 3 months.

To reheat: Defrost overnight in the refrigerator. When you're ready to serve the ragù, add the defrosted or still frozen cubes to a saucepan and warm over a low-medium heat until fully defrosted and piping hot. Let the ragù cool before serving with your favourite carb companion.

NOTE

If you have time, leave the sauce to simmer gently over a low heat for up to 1 hour so the flavours can really intensify.

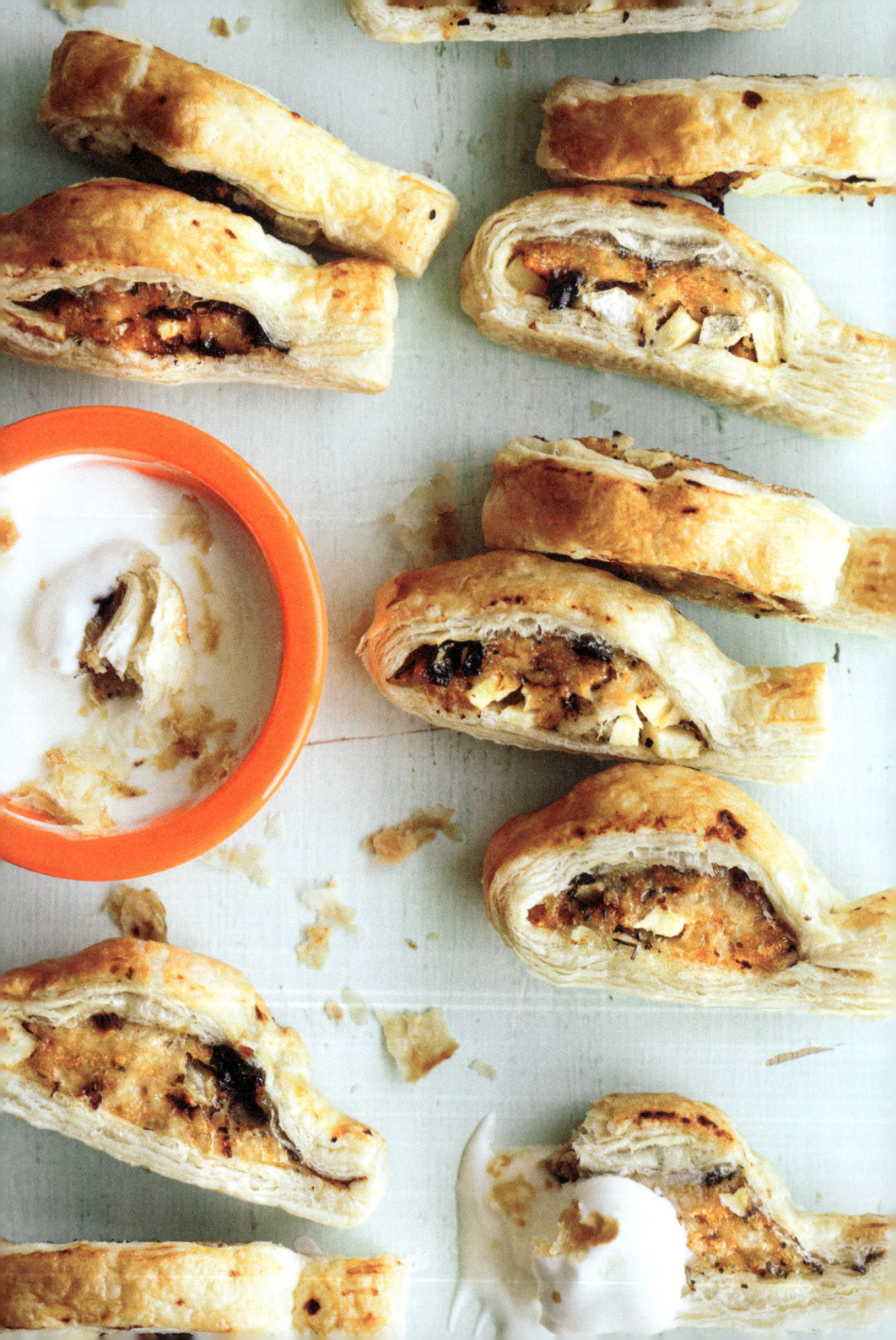

MINI FRUITY CHICKEN ROLLS

|||||||||||||||||||||||||||||||||||||||||||||||||||||||||||||||||||||||||||||||||||||||||||||||||

These delectable, flaky delights rival the classic salt-laden pork sausage rolls. Ideal for lunch or effortless teas, they are infused with delightful apple and prune notes.

Prep + cook time: **25 mins**

MAKES 48 PORTIONS

500g (1lb 2oz/generous 2 cups) minced (ground) chicken
1 onion, finely diced
2 apples, peeled and finely diced
40g (1½oz/¼ cup) pitted prunes, finely diced
2 teaspoons dried rosemary
150g (5oz/1⅔ cup) dried breadcrumbs
2 ready-rolled puff pastry sheets
1 medium egg, beaten

Allergy swaps: Swap the egg for 2 teaspoons full-fat milk or vegetable oil. Swap the puff pastry for a gluten-free variety, and swap the breadcrumbs for gluten-free breadcrumbs, crushed gluten-free cornflakes or puffed rice cereal.

1. Preheat the oven to 240°C/220°C fan/475°F/Gas mark 9, and line 2 baking trays (sheet pans) with baking parchment.
2. In a large bowl, combine the minced chicken, onion, apples, prunes, rosemary and dried breadcrumbs.
3. Unroll the puff pastry sheets and slice them in half lengthways to create 4 long strips.
4. Scoop out a quarter of the chicken mix, form it into a sausage shape and place it in the centre of a sheet of pastry, leaving a 1cm (½in) border. Repeat with the remaining chicken mix and pastry sheets.
5. Brush the borders of the pastry with the egg wash, then roll the long edges of the pastry tightly over the sausage. Press gently to secure it. Turn the roll so you end up with the seam underneath.
6. Slice off any extra pastry at the ends and then cut each roll into 2cm (¾in) pieces, making 12 mini chicken rolls (48 in total).
7. Place the mini rolls on the baking tray and brush with more egg wash. Bake for 15 minutes, or until golden, crisp and cooked through.
8. Serve once cooled, or wrap and freeze for up to 3 months.

To reheat: Defrost at room temperature for 1–2 hours, or overnight in the refrigerator. Serve cold, or heat in the microwave for 15 seconds per roll. Alternatively, preheat the oven to 200°C/180°C fan/400°F/Gas mark 6, cover the rolls with foil and bake for 15–20 minutes until cooked through. Let the rolls cool before serving.

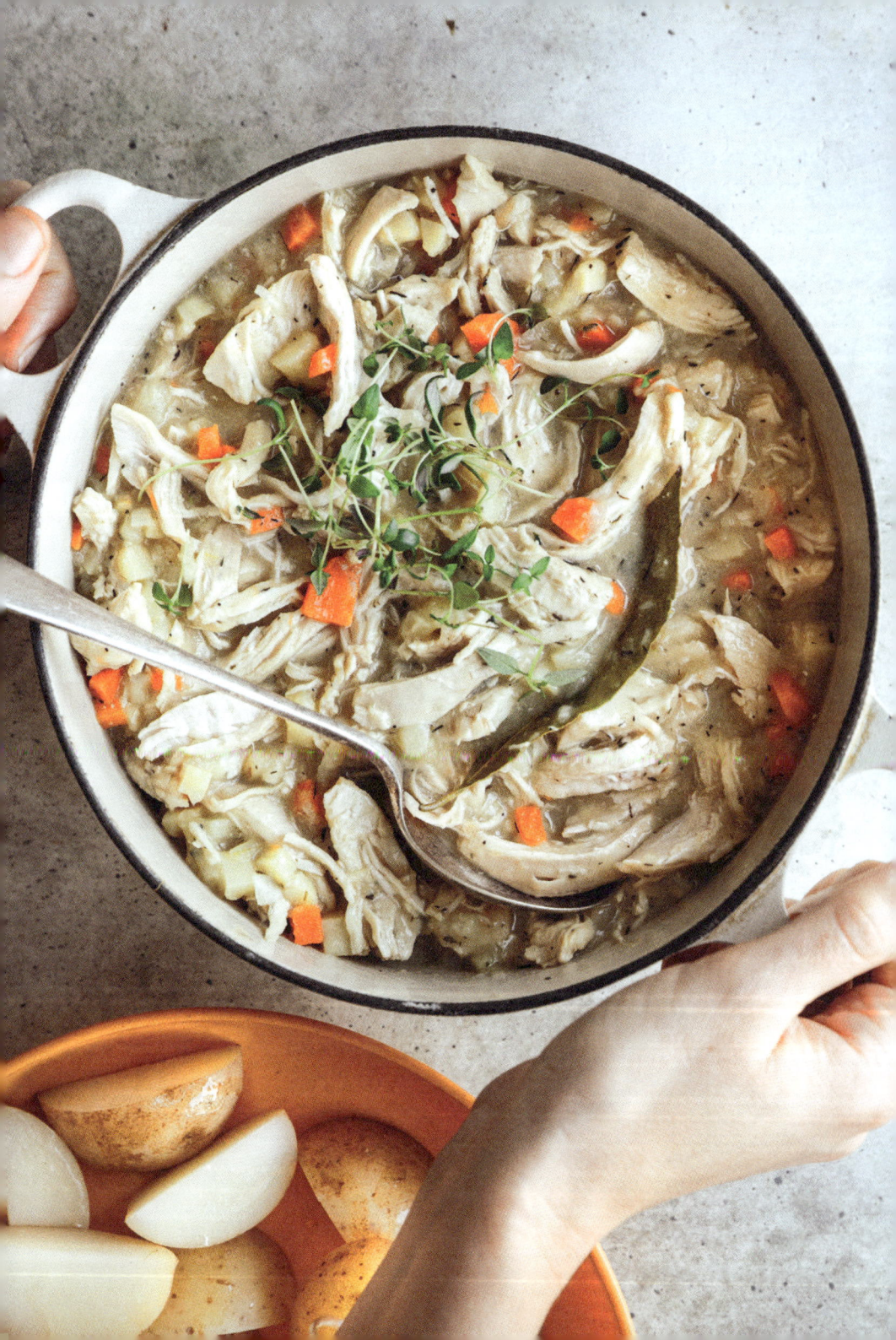

SERIOUSLY GOOD SHREDDED CHICKEN STEW

||||||||||||||||||||||||||||||||||||||||||||||||||||||||||||||||||||||||||||||||||||||||||||||||||||||||||||||||||||||

Picture this: a pot bubbling with moreish shredded chicken, a treasure trove of hearty goodness tailor-made for little hands to grasp. It's not just a recipe; it's a dance of flavours, a medley of textures and a celebration of the heartwarming moments shared around the table.

Prep + cook time: **25 mins**

MAKES 8–10 PORTIONS

400g (14oz) new potatoes, sliced into quarters
1 tablespoon vegetable oil
1 carrot, very finely diced
1 parsnip, very finely diced
1 onion, very finely diced
500g (1lb 2oz) chicken breasts, each sliced into 4 equal chunks
2 tablespoons plain (all-purpose) flour
600ml (20fl oz/2½ cups) low-salt chicken stock (broth)
2 teaspoons dried thyme
1 bay leaf

Allergy swaps: Swap the flour for gluten-free.

1. Set a large saucepan of water on the hob to boil over a medium heat. Once bubbling, add the potatoes and simmer for 8–10 minutes until tender, then drain and set aside.
2. In the meantime, heat the oil in a large saucepan over a high heat and fry the carrot, parsnip, onion and chicken for 3 minutes.
3. Add the flour and stir until the vegetables and chicken are well coated.
4. Add the chicken stock, thyme and bay leaf, and cook over a high heat for 12 minutes.
5. Turn off the heat and remove the chicken (ensuring it is fully cooked through), shred it with two forks and then stir it back into the stew alongside the cooked new potatoes.
6. Let the stew cool, then portion it into freezer-safe containers and freeze for up to 3 months.

To reheat: Defrost overnight in the refrigerator. Once you're ready to serve, add the stew to a saucepan and warm over a medium heat until piping hot. Let the stew cool before serving.

SUPERSIZED STROGANOFF

Indulge in the ultimate comfort food experience with this supersized stroganoff! With tender chicken, aromatic sweet paprika, peppery parsley and just a touch of zesty Dijon mustard, it's a flavour-packed delight for the whole family to savour. My convenient make-ahead freezing method means you'll always have delicious portions ready for a stress-free supper.

Prep + cook time: **20 mins**

MAKES 8–10 PORTIONS

2 teaspoons vegetable oil
2 large onions, finely diced
1kg (2lb 3oz) chicken
   breasts, sliced
3 teaspoons minced garlic
2 teaspoons sweet
   smoked paprika
2 teaspoons dried parsley
1 litre (34fl oz/4 cups)
   chicken stock (broth)
8 teaspoons Dijon
   mustard
400g (14oz/1¾ cups)
   cream cheese

1. Heat the oil in a large saucepan over a medium-high heat and fry the onion for 5 minutes until softened.
2. Add the sliced chicken and fry for 5 minutes until cooked through.
3. Add the garlic, smoked paprika and parsley and stir through for 1 minute.
4. Add the stock and mustard, then cook for another 5 minutes.
5. Finally, turn off the heat and stir through the cream cheese to create a creamy sauce.
6. Let the stroganoff cool, then portion it into large ice-cube trays or freezer-safe containers and freeze for up to 3 months.

To reheat: Defrost overnight in the refrigerator. When you're ready to serve, add the stroganoff to a saucepan and warm slowly, to avoid it curdling, over a low heat until piping hot. Let the stroganoff cool before serving.

Allergy swaps: For a dairy allergy, swap the cream cheese for a dairy-free soft cheese.

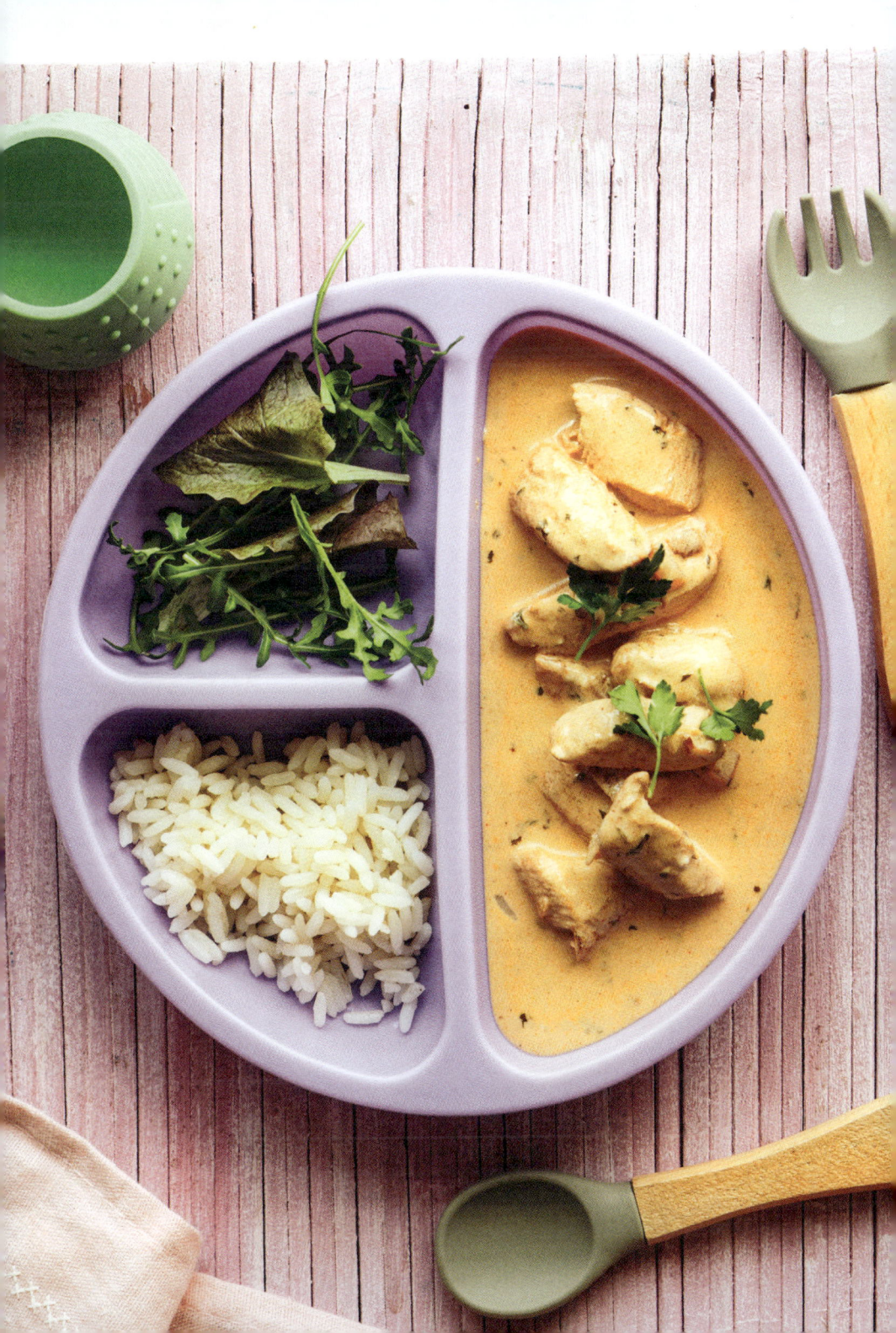

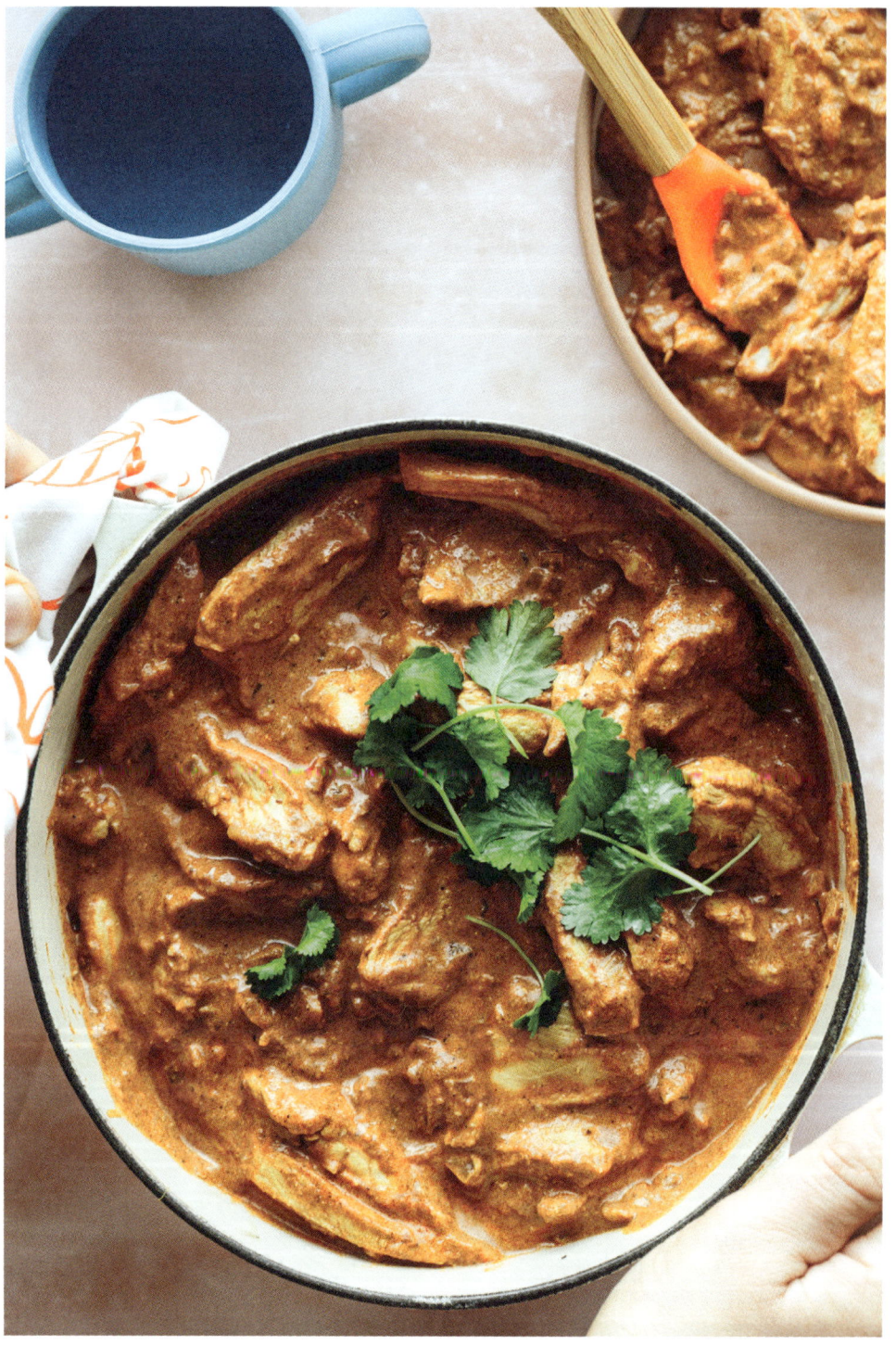

BIG BATCH BUTTER CHICKEN

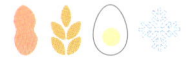

||||||||||||||||||||||||||||||||||||||||||||||||||||||||||||||||||||||||||||||||||||||||||||||||||||

This butter chicken could rival a takeaway, and what's more, it only takes 15 minutes to prepare. It's deliciously creamy with notes of fragrant spice, making it the perfect introduction to a little heat. Serve with fluffy rice and soft strips of warm naan bread.

Prep + cook time: **20 mins**

MAKES 8–10 PORTIONS

1 teaspoon vegetable oil
2 onions, finely diced
4 teaspoons minced garlic
1kg (2lb 3oz) chicken breasts, sliced
8 tablespoons tomato purée (paste)
2 tablespoons brown sugar (optional)
2 tablespoons garam masala
2 teaspoons mild chilli powder
2 teaspoons ground cumin
500ml (17fl oz/2 cups) full-fat natural yoghurt

1. Heat the oil in a large saucepan over a medium heat and fry the onion for 4 minutes until softened.
2. Add the garlic, stirring consistently for 1 minute.
3. Add the chicken and fry for 5 minutes until fully cooked through.
4. Add the tomato purée, brown sugar (if using) and spices and cook for another 5 minutes.
5. Turn off the heat and stir through the yoghurt.
6. Let the curry cool, then portion it into large ice-cube trays or freezer-safe containers and freeze for up to 3 months.

To reheat: Defrost overnight in the refrigerator. When you're ready to serve, add the curry to a saucepan and warm over a medium heat until piping hot. Let the curry cool before serving.

Allergy swaps: For a dairy allergy, swap the yoghurt for soya, coconut or oat yoghurt.

RESOURCES

www.babyledweaningcourse.co.uk

www.allergyuk.org/types-of-allergies/food-allergy/

www.allergyuk.org/resources/weaning-support-pack/

www.nhs.uk/conditions/baby/weaning-and-feeding/food-allergies-in-babies-and-young-children/

www.anaphylaxis.org.uk/living-with-serious-allergies/infant-weaning/

www.nhs.uk/start4life/

www.bda.uk.com/resource/complementary-feeding-weaning.html

REFERENCES

Boswell, N. (July 2021) 'Complementary Feeding Methods – A Review of the Benefits and Risks', *International Journal of Environmental Research and Public Health.*

Brown, A., Jones, S. and Rowan, H. (2017). 'Baby-Led Weaning: The Evidence to Date', *Current Nutrition Reports.*

Townsend, E. and Pitchford N. J. (2012) 'Baby knows best? The impact of weaning style on food preferences and body mass index in early childhood in a case-controlled sample', *BMJ Open.*

ACKNOWLEDGEMENTS

This book has been simmering within me for years, but it wouldn't have been possible without the unwavering support of some truly remarkable individuals.

First and foremost, to my beautiful daughter, **Annabelle** – none of this would be a reality without you. Thank you from the bottom of my heart. I'm so truly proud of you. Your drive, zest for life and creativity fuel me every day. I am deeply grateful for your belief in me.

To my delightful twins, **Alex** and **Oliver** – thank you for your boundless love and patience, even at your tender age. Your infectious joy brightens each day, and though you may prefer *Tabby McTat* for now, I hope one day you'll read this and understand the immense inspiration you've been to me.

To **Steve** – your love and support have sustained me through moments of doubt. Thank you for being my rock, for taste-testing every recipe without complaint and for your invaluable help with the children, enabling me to pour my heart into this book.

To **Mum** and **Dad** – your unwavering support has meant the world to me: thank you for always believing in me and my creative endeavours. I hope I've made you proud.

To **Bob** and **Ro** – your support and encouragement have been indispensable. Without you, this dream would have remained just that – a dream.

To **Debbie** – your belief in my potential at college has propelled me forward. Your encouragement has been a driving force behind my achievements, and for that, I am truly grateful.

To **Nicole** – your belief in me and this project has been a beacon of encouragement. I am deeply grateful for the incredible opportunity you've given me.

To **Lucy K** – your support and guidance have been instrumental in shaping this book. Your wealth of knowledge has illuminated every step of the journey, and I am profoundly thankful for your wisdom.

To **Lucy U** – thank you for your boundless support and expertise, which have elevated this project to new heights. Your invaluable contributions have enriched the book, making it truly exceptional.

To all my social media followers – thank you for embracing my authenticity and joining me on this journey of food and weaning. Your support has meant everything.

And to you, dear reader – thank you for choosing to be a part of this. Your trust in me to support you and your little one fills me with gratitude beyond words.

Thank you from the bottom of my heart.

INDEX

First published in Great Britain in 2024 by
Greenfinch
An imprint of Quercus Editions Ltd
Carmelite House
50 Victoria Embankment
London
EC4Y 0DZ

An Hachette UK company

A CIP catalogue record for this book is available
from the British Library.

HB ISBN 978-1-52943-638-9
eBook ISBN 978-1-52943-639-6

10 9 8 7 6 5 4 3 2 1

Commissioning Editor: Nicole Thomas
Project Editor: Lucy Kingett
Designer: Clare Sivell
Photography and prop styling: Kimberly Espinel
Food styling: Holly Cowgill

Printed and bound in Croatia by Denona

Papers used by Greenfinch are from well-managed forests
and other responsible sources.